Puppy Owner's Veterinary Care Book

James DeBitetto, D.V.M.

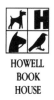

HOWELL
BOOK
HOUSE

Howell Book House
MACMILLAN
A Simon & Schuster-Macmillan Company
1633 Broadway
New York, NY 10019

Library of Congress Cataloging-in-Publication Data

DeBitetto, James.
    The puppy owner's veterinary care book/James DeBitetto.
       p.   cm.
    Includes bibliographical references and index.
    ISBN 0-87605-786-5
    1. Puppies—Diseases—Handbooks, manuals, etc. 2. Puppies—Health—
        Handbooks, manuals, etc. 3. Veterinary pediatrics—Handbooks,
        manuals,
        etc. I. Title.
        SF991.D54   1995
        636.7'089892—dc20   94-45975
                                         CIP

ISBN: 0-87605-786-5

Manufactured in the United States of America
10 9 8 7 6 5 4 3 2 1

Photos and medical illustrations by Dr. James DeBitetto unless otherwise credited.

Book Design by designLab.

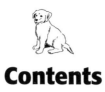

Contents

Acknowledgments

I find myself yet again thanking people for their help on a puppy book. I must thank Dominique DeVito for her skillful editing and all her energy in making this book for puppy owners a one of a kind, and a "must have." I'd like to again thank my publisher, Sean Frawley and all the wonderful people at Howell Book House for being supportive and a pleasure to work with. Next, I'd like to thank the best staff any veterinarian could ever hope for at Country Home Veterinary Clinic: Katie, Penny, Jacqueline and Donna. Thank you again for your patience for putting up with me for the two years this book was in production. A special thanks to my groomer, Pam Koerner, for her help in the grooming section and the use of her beautiful puppies for a few photo shoots. She truly has a wealth of knowledge in all aspects of the dog world.

A sincere thanks to Arlene Oraby—a dear friend, for her enormous help with editing the manuscript, and for allowing me to photograph her beautiful Great Pyrenees puppies. I'd like to thank a long-time colleague and friend, Dr. Marjorie Neaderland, for donating her slides of eye disorders, and her help as veterinary ophthalmologist. A warm thanks to Dr. Dwight D. Bowman and his assistant Ms. Marguerite Frongillo at the College of Veterinary Medicine at Cornell University for supplying pictures of parasites and bugs.

I'd like to thank the late Dr. Edward Grano, Jr., whom I trained under for so many years, for giving me the guidance and compassion needed to be a true veterinarian. And to all my clients who let me photograph their puppies and whose good questions and concerns prompted me to write this book.

Perhaps most of all, I'd like to thank my parents and family for their support through the years. A special thanks to my brother, Bob, for all his help with the legal work and contacts. With all my heart, I'd like to thank my wife, Donna, for without her, none of the last ten years would have been possible. She has helped me in every aspect of my life, including this book; I love her so. And lastly, to my best friend, Myles, my black Labrador Retriever, who has taught me the power of perseverance.

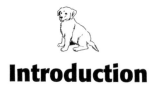

Introduction

Congratulations on your new puppy! If you're like so many new puppy owners, you must be thrilled, excited, and perhaps a bit overwhelmed. Don't worry, that's normal. Most new parents are. After all, a new puppy is a lot like a baby, only a bit furrier.

The concerns, questions, problems, and joys involved in beecoming the owner of a new puppy are very similar to those facing the parents of a new baby. And just as new parents turn to first-year baby-care books, new puppy owners should have a resource for complete state-of-the-art information on puppy health care. Why should they be forced to read a book about adult dog care? Puppy pediatrics is very different from adult dog health care.

The importance of early health care can't be stressed enough. "Well visits" are now the emphasis in baby health care. A well visit is when the baby is brought in for preventive health care before he or she gets sick. This concept is not new in veterinary medicine. We have been emphasizing well-puppy care for years with regular, early veterinary visits and vaccination protocols. Veterinarians have been vaccinating and thwarting disease in young puppies for decades. Early detection means early treatment, with a better chance of a speedy recovery. In fact, you could say veterinarians invented the concept of well visits. *It only makes sense that the key to better health is early disease detection and prevention.*

This book is the most comprehensive puppy-care book in print. Topics cover all health issues that could arise during a puppy's first year of life, much of which continues to be applicable as a puppy grows, because a great deal of the information spans beyond the first year. I detail topics that include birth defects; vaccinations; parasites; preventive health maintenance of ears, eyes, teeth and coat; nutrition and feeding; home remedies and holistic alternatives; household dangers; first aid and pediatrics.

The best way to use this book is as a general health guide. You can learn more about puppy health topics, or you can use the information for reference. If your veterinarian finds something wrong with your puppy, you can go home and look up the ailment. But let me make one thing clear: *This book is in no way a substitute for your veterinarian.* It is crucial that you develop a good relationship with your veterinarian so that he or she can keep your new best friend happy and healthy. Work with your vet. Try to find one who respects a preventive health approach. Together, you should enjoy many years of a healthy, happy puppy. Healthy puppies grow into healthy adult dogs. The best compliment you can give your veterinarian years down the road is, "You know, Doc, even though my dog is seven years old, he still acts like a puppy. Thanks to you!"

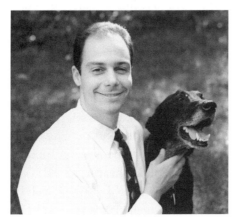

Dr. James DeBitetto and Myles.
Donna DeBitetto.

First Aid Kit for Puppies

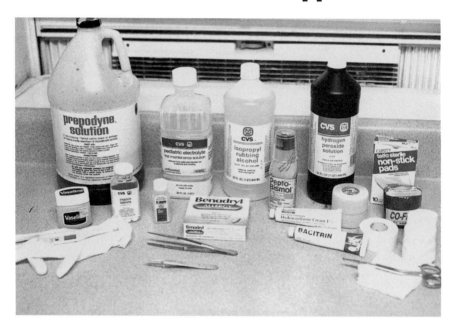

Ace Bandage
Adult Aspirin (Buffered or
enteric coated)
Antibiotic Skin Ointment
Antihistamine Tablets
Baby Aspirin
Bandage Scissors
Bismuth Anti-diarrhea Medication
Gauze, 2" Rolls and 2"×2" Squares
Hydrocortisone Skin Ointment

Hydrogen Peroxide
Latex Exam Gloves
Medical Tape (White), 1" Roll
Non-stick Pads
Pediatric Electrolyte Oral Solution
Petroleum Jelly (White)
Povidone Antiseptic Solution
Rectal Thermometer
Rubbing Alcohol
Tweezers

Chapter 1

Congenital and Inherited Defects

As miraculous and splendid as nature is in its ability to reproduce and propagate the species, one really must marvel at how complicated the reproductive process is, and that it works as often as it does. Ask any dog breeder how frustrating and complex breeding can be—from timing the ovulation of the bitch during her heat cycle with successful natural breeding or artificial insemination, to an uneventful whelping and a healthy litter of puppies.

The joy of birth can easily be spoiled with any number of mishaps, none as devastating as a puppy with a birth defect. Some are serious, others are not. This chapter will cover all the common inherited (meaning genetically passed on) and congenital (meaning present at birth) defects. We will try to give you an idea of their severity, when they can be detected, and by whom; whether you should seek immediate medical care for your puppy or wait; and a forecast as to the outcome of the illness—that is, its *prognosis*.

What a Prognosis Means

When a health professional gives his or her assessment or prediction of a particular condition, it is called a prognosis. This is a grading system to give the patient an idea of how serious the problem or disease is and how good the chances of a complete recovery are. Think of it as a medical forecast. The following is the traditional rating system:

Excellent Prognosis. This means that the condition or disease is not serious at all and the likelihood of a complete recovery is almost certain. An example of this would be a mild dermatitis or skin irritation.

Good Prognosis. This means that the condition or disease is not serious but should not be ignored. Some medical treatment may be needed, but the likelihood of a complete recovery is good. Examples of this would be either a more severe dermatitis or an otitis externa (outer ear infection).

Fair Prognosis. This means that the condition or disease warrants medical attention promptly. Medical treatment is always required and may be prolonged. Despite the ominous tone of this prognosis, the outcome is generally favorable. Recovery is expected, if not complete. These conditions should be taken seriously, and follow-up medical attention may be needed. An example of this would be a collapsing trachea (described later in this chapter).

Guarded Prognosis. These conditions have the potential of becoming serious. In other words, the outcome could go either way. These cases must be treated promptly and aggressively. Follow-ups are always needed to assess the effectiveness of the treatment. An example of this would be a case of persistent bronchitis.

Poor Prognosis. These conditions or diseases are serious. The animal is usually debilitated or compromised in some way. Attempts at treatment may help but are not guaranteed. These conditions are usually chronic or are a result of acute trauma. Owners given a poor prognosis for their pet should seek a second opinion if they have any reservations about care being given or a lack of communication with the veterinarian. Many owners choose euthanasia when given a poor prognosis. Examples of conditions that may carry a poor prognosis are certain cancers, heart failure, kidney failure, hepatitis, terminal viral diseases, and severe trauma with shock.

Grave Prognosis. As the name implies, the conditions and diseases that give a grave prognosis are terminal. There is very little hope for these patients, and modern medicine has little to offer. Most owners resign themselves to the fate of their pet and start to prepare for the final arrangements. Examples of this would be end-stage heart disease or heart failure.

Defects Noticed at Birth

This section provides an alphabetical list of congenital defects that the breeder usually notices within a few days of birth. Some are more serious than others. We mention when a veterinarian is needed to make the diagnosis, because many of these are not easy to spot at first.

Cleft Palate and Harelip

During the embryonic development of the fetus, two folds of tissue come together to form the bones of the roof of the mouth, or palate. If something interrupts this process, there will be a gap or cleft in the roof of the mouth. This gap can range from a few millimeters to a centimeter. These clefts are usually noticed immediately after birth by the breeder. Simple examination of the roof of the mouth will reveal the opening. The consequences of this can be severe. If the cleft is small, it can close on its own, usually within a month or two. However, only a small percentage of clefts do. More commonly, the cleft is too large to close naturally, and, as the newborn nurses, milk is sucked from the mouth into the nasal passages and then is inhaled into the lungs, where it starts an aspiration pneumonia.

Many puppies with this affliction are euthanized; therefore the prognosis is *guarded*. Occasionally, if the neonate survives to two or three months of age, surgical correction can be attempted. Since cleft palates are inherited from the dam or sire, most breeders will not breed the same pair of dogs again. There appears to be more of a predilection in the breeds with short "pushed-in" faces, such as the Pekingese, the Bulldog and the Boston Terrier. Occasionally a cleft palate occurs together with a cleft lip (also known as a harelip).

Hermaphrodites, or Intersexing

One of the joys of having a new litter of puppies is to try to determine how many males and females there are—what we call "sexing the litter." Occasionally, however, a specific neonate cannot be sexed. This is usually because it is neither a male nor a female but a cross between the two. The external genitals do not look like a normal male's or female's. What's more, internally these puppies are usually abnormal as well, with males having ovaries inside or females having testicles instead of ovaries. A veterinarian is usually needed to make this differentiation. No specific treatment is needed. However, cosmetic corrective surgery to make the dog's appearance more normal can be performed. These puppies are sterile and cannot be bred. Occasionally this defect is associated with other defects of the urogenital system, so a thorough examination by a veterinarian is needed. Barring any other complications, hermaphrodites generally lead normal lives (except they cannot be used for breeding), and the prognosis is *good*.

Imperforate Anus

This is a condition characterized by the absence of an anal opening. The word "imperforate" means "no opening." Can you imagine being born without an anus? The breeder usually notices within a day or so because there is no defecation or feces from this puppy. Upon closer inspection of the rectal area, the breeder finds that the puppy has no anus. The backup of feces causes distention of the colon first, then of the small intestine. In actuality, there are several different types of imperforate anus. In some instances, the puppy actually has no anus, as has just been described, which is the most common case. A variation of this condition occurs when a puppy apparently does have an anal opening but its rectum is closed less than an inch inside, like a dead-end tube. This condition is detected when the breeder or veterinarian tries to pass a rectal thermometer up the puppy's rectum. Treatment of this defect is to open the anus surgically. There is no breed predilection; however, females seem to be more prone to this condition, and it is often associated with other malformations of the anovaginal area, as described in the next section under "Anovaginal Fistulae." The prognosis is *fair* to *good*, depending on which form of the defect is present and whether corrective surgery is successful.

Skeletal Defects

Puppies can be born with a variety of skeletal deformities. Some are serious, whereas others are merely inconvenient. The following four are the most common.

Hydrocephalus. This is commonly called "water on the brain," and that pretty much sums it up. This condition is caused by cerebral spinal fluid buildup between the skull bone plates and the brain and the spinal tissue, due to a reduced outflow. The puppy has an enlarged head at birth. The breeds with the highest incidence of this condition are the Maltese, Yorkshire Terrier, Bulldog, Chihuahua, Pekingese, Toy Poodle and Lhasa Apso. Symptoms include neurological disturbances, circling, seizures, head pressing and aimless crawling. Most of these cases do not need treatment. Occasionally, however, this fluid must be drained off the brain to relieve the pressure. The prognosis for the mild to moderate cases is *fair* to *good*. For the severe cases, the prognosis is *guarded*, because permanent brain damage can result in having to euthanize the puppy.

Open Fontanel. The fontanel is the area at the center of the top of the skull where the three bone plates come together during fetal development to form the top of the skull. In a small percentage of neonates, these bone plates never fully come together and fuse, leaving a hole in the center. This is a common occurrence and should not be of too much concern. Care should be taken not to apply too much pressure on the top of the puppy's head until the plates fuse at about four weeks of age. Certain breeds are more prone to this condition. They are the same breeds that have a high incidence of hydrocephalus, as described under that heading. Perhaps the most common breed is the Chihuahua. No treatment is needed, and the prognosis is *good*. There doesn't seem to be a sex predilection.

Spina Bifida. The most common spinal deformity seen in newborn puppies is called *spina bifida*. This is when the spinal column of the lower lumbar, or back, which is a column of embryonic tissue, never closes properly but remains open at birth. This defect is terribly debilitating due to the deformity of the lower spine. Puppies show paralysis of the hind legs, urinary bladder and rectum. The condition is inherited from either parent and usually warrants immediate euthanasia of the puppy. Therefore, the prognosis is *grave*. The novice breeder should immediately consult with a veterinarian if a puppy is born with an opening along the lower spinal column. There is no breed or sex predilection for this condition.

Swimmers (Flat Puppy Syndrome). This is a deformity of the chest wall and sternum (breast plate) of newborn puppies. This deformity causes the newborn to paddle and "swim" without being able to sit up. The puppy's breathing patterns are irregular and can be distressed. If the puppy survives the initial few weeks, it can often compensate for its weakness and start to stand. The prognosis is *guarded* to *fair*.

Skin Disorders

Newborns can be born with a variety of skin afflictions. Some are true defects of the skin; others are acquired during transport through the birth canal or even while the puppy is still in the uterus (*in utero*). Both are described here.

Acquired Skin Diseases of Newborns. These are usually either bacterial or fungal. The most common bacterial infections of the skin are *Staphylococcus* and *Streptococcus* bacteria. They are often found in the vaginal tract of the bitch. The fetus is infected either *in utero* (inside the uterus) or during the passage through the vaginal canal. The skin appears yellow to tan in color. Pustules (whiteheads) can be seen on the trunk of the body; these lesions crust and ooze a pus discharge.

Fungal infections are also contracted *in utero*, as yeast (the budding form of fungus) is also a common inhabitant of the vaginal tract. They both appear as blotches or areas of skin that are discolored, molted or crusted or which contain bleeding plaques. The two most common skin fungal agents are *Candida albicans* and *Microsporum* (commonly known as ringworm). A veterinarian is needed to differentiate between the two types. Treatments with antibiotics, anti-fungal drugs and medicated sponge baths (usually with an organic iodine solution) are very effective. Therefore, the prognosis is usually *good*. There is no breed or sex predilection for this condition.

Hypotrichosis. A puppy that is born with this inherited skin defect has only remnants of hair follicles, which are incapable of growing hair. The result is a hairless dog. Hypotrichosis can occur in certain color varieties of dogs, such as the blue or tan Doberman Pinscher or the silver Toy Poodle. This defect is expected in certain breeds such as the Chinese Crested and Mexican Hairless. Obviously, in those breeds that are bred for this trait, it is considered normal. The experienced breeder can usually pick these puppies out within a few weeks of whelping. The prognosis is *good*, and the only treatment necessary is for accompanying seborrhea.

Rubber Puppy Syndrome. As the name implies, the skin of these puppies is rubbery and elastic. The scientific name for this condition is Ehlers-Danlos syndrome. The breeds reported with this are the Springer Spaniel, Beagle, Boxer, German Shepherd, Greyhound, Dachshund and St. Bernard. The skin is immediately noted as tissue-paper thin and easily torn. There is no treatment other than being very careful not to tear or rip the skin, and the prognosis is *guarded* to *fair*.

Stillborn

This condition is simply defined as a puppy that is born dead. There are many reasons why puppies are stillborn, including poor oxygenation of the fetal blood during whelping; the puppy being caught in the pelvic birth canal for too long; numerous infectious diseases such as *Escherichia coli*, *Streptococcus*, *Brucella*, and *Chlamydia* or *Mycoplasma* bacteria; and severe internal defects such as heart abnormalities that would only be discovered upon autopsy. Obviously, the prognosis of this condition is *grave*.

Most novice breeders can easily tell when a puppy is deceased, by its lack of movement and breathing. As sad as this is, there should always be an inquiry into the cause of death, as it may be prevented in the next breeding, or it may be a symptom of a problem with the bitch. There is no breed or sex predilection for this condition. Your veterinarian should always be consulted about a stillborn puppy, as he or she would most likely want to determine the cause of death via autopsy and bacterial cultures. Environmental factors such as hypothermia (chilling), inadequate nursing or suckling reflex, accidental crushing by the dam, insufficient milk production by the dam or rejection by the dam are also causes of neonatal death, but these problems are not congenital defects.

Umbilical and Inguinal Hernias

Occasionally, puppies are born with a hole either in their abdominal wall in the area of the navel (called the *umbilicus*), or in the groin (scientifically know as the *inguinal* area). In the case of the umbilical hernia, the problem is either genetic or because the bitch chewed the umbilical cord too short. To avoid umbilical herniation, there should be a minimum of 1 to 1¹/₂ inches of umbilicus remaining on the puppy's stomach. This is good to know if you are involved in cutting the umbilical cords. The cause of the inguinal hernia is usually genetic.

The first thing noticed is a swelling either of the abdominal wall at the belly button for the umbilical hernia, or in the groin area for the inguinal, respectively. Neither is a life-threatening condition in the neonate. As the puppy grows and becomes more active, a loop of bowel may fall into the hole in the abdominal wall and strangulate itself, which could be dangerous. Therefore, your veterinarian has to assess whether the hernia is large enough to warrant surgical closure when the puppy is of age (usually when it is spayed or neutered at six months). Abdominal fat causes the swelling or bulge at the hernia site. If you are able to push the fat back inside the belly, then the hernia is classified as "reducible." If you cannot push the fat back inside, then it is classified as "non-reducible." The non-reducible hernias carry a better prognosis and seldom require surgery.

The prognosis of congenital hernia is *fair* to *good*. There is no predilection for this condition, but male puppies are more prone to getting the inguinal hernia because they naturally have an opening in the lower body wall where the testicles descend into the scrotum. If this opening doesn't close in time (usually by four to six weeks of age), an inguinal hernia may result.

Defects Noticed by Eight Weeks of Age

Many congenital conditions may not show up at birth but usually do by eight weeks—the age at which a puppy is most likely to be bought. This section contains an alphabetical list of the most common birth defects that can be detected during the first visit to the vet, and he or she should be on the lookout for them. There is nothing wrong with your asking, "Doc, do you see any birth defects I should be concerned about?"

Anovaginal Fistulae

This condition is related to the imperforate anus, as described in the previous section. In this case, a direct connection or opening exists between the vagina and the rectum. This is serious because the potential is great for the feces to contaminate the vaginal tract and cause a variety of vaginal and uterus infections. Therefore, this defect is surgically corrected when the puppy is older (around sixteen weeks old). A veterinarian is usually needed to make the diagnosis. Although this defect is present at birth, a close examination of the genitals may not be done until the puppy is several weeks old. Obviously, this condition affects only females. There doesn't appear to be any breed predilection. Treatment is surgical closure of the opening when the puppy is of age to undergo anesthesia. With surgery, the prognosis is generally *good*. The puppy is always treated with antibiotics to help reduce the chance of vaginal and uterine infections.

Dental Defects

Teeth are one of the first things most veterinarians check for at an eight-week exam. Breeders are especially concerned about the bite of the puppy and the health of the deciduous (puppy) teeth. Although all these baby teeth will fall out at four to six months and be replaced with permanent adult teeth, they are an important predictor as to the health of the permanent dentition. Poor bites are ones that have a malocclusion—that is, when the top and bottom rows of teeth do not line up properly. Other than malocclusion, a poor bite can be defined as having missing teeth, too many teeth, teeth in the wrong position, or unhealthy teeth. Following is an alphabetical list of the most common dental defects.

> *Absence of Teeth*. This inherited condition is seen in specific breeds such as the Collie and the Doberman Pinscher, and is called *anodontia*. It can range from having only a few teeth missing, such as the incisors or a premolar, to having entire rows of teeth missing. By the time a puppy is eight weeks of age, all its puppy teeth should have cut their way through the gum line. Sometimes, however, a puppy has a normal set of deciduous teeth but no permanent teeth that follow. These poor puppies then become toothless adults. This form of anodontia is perhaps the most severe; even so, the prognosis is *good*, as dogs can lead a normal life without any teeth. They can be fed soft and canned foods, but they should not be bred, as this trait is hereditary. There is no treatment for anodontia, and there is no sex predilection.

> *Enamel Defects*. The enamel is the white, hard coating of teeth. It is the hardest material in the body. The enamel is essential in maintaining tooth health. If, during the development of the tooth from its tooth bud, certain factors are present, faulty enamel can result. Instead of enamel that is white, smooth and impermeable, the defective enamel is thin, brown and soft. This ultimately leads to tooth loss. There doesn't

seem to be any genetic basis for this condition. Environmental factors play more of a role, such as whether the dam had any viral diseases during her pregnancy or whether the puppy was given any antibiotics in the tetracycline family. Again, the prognosis is *good*, as this condition is never life-threatening. It can be disastrous, however, for a show dog's career. Practically speaking, no treatment is available for this problem. But with advances in veterinary dentistry, such as bonding, minor enamel defects can be corrected. No specific breed or sex is prone to this condition.

Overshot and Undershot Jaw. These are lay terms for bad bites, and both are inherited defects that run in certain families. Overshot jaw (scientifically called *brachygnathism*) is when the upper jaw is longer than and extends past the lower jaw. Breeds most susceptible are those with longer muzzles, such as the Collie, Shetland Sheepdog, Greyhound and others. Undershot jaw (scientifically called *prognathism*) is when the lower jaw is longer than or extends past the upper jaw. The breeds most likely to be afflicted are the short-faced ones, such as the Pug, Pekingese, Bulldog, Boston Terrier and Lhasa Apso. There is no treatment for either condition, as it is more cosmetic than functionally wrong. Of course, the defects are breeding faults and these dogs should not be bred. The prognosis is *good*, because these jaw defects don't seem to interfere with the dog's ability to eat.

Supernumerary Teeth. This is a common defect where there are more teeth than normal. An extra tooth bud emerges, resulting in an extra tooth squeezed between two normal ones. The extra tooth is often smaller than normal and can push the normal teeth aside, causing a poor alignment. Therefore, the treatment is to extract the extra tooth so that it doesn't interfere with the normal dentition. Supernumerary teeth can be seen in almost all breeds and both sexes. The prognosis is always *good*.

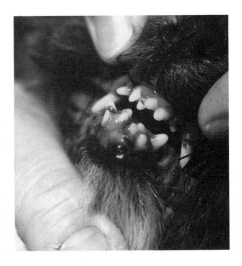

An example of supernumerary teeth, or extra teeth growing in and squeezing the others.

Split or Twin Crown. In this developmental problem, the tooth bud either splits or fuses with another tooth bud during development of a puppy tooth. The result is a tooth, usually an incisor, that looks as if it were split down the center. Actually, two crowns are sharing one root. This can also happen in adult teeth. There is no breed predilection, and since it is only a cosmetic concern, the prognosis is *good*.

Digestive Defects

Puppies have a wide variety of gastrointestinal problems, but most are due to simple factors such as overeating, eating inappropriate things, internal parasites, and so on. These problems are covered in Chapter 6, "Puppy Pediatrics." This section concentrates on congenital defects of the intestinal tract. Following are descriptions of the four most common digestive defects.

Dysphagia. This term means "difficulty in swallowing." During the eating process, food is first chewed, then swallowed. Swallowing is a complex coordinated function of muscle contractions. If any part of this effort goes awry, swallowing doesn't happen. The cause of dysphagia is usually a malfunction of the nerves controlling the tongue or larynx. The first symptom the breeder notices is food falling out of the puppy's mouth during eating. Besides the physical evidence, contrast radiographs can demonstrate the location of the problem. Surgical treatments have been tried with limited success. Feeding tubes are sometimes used to deliver the food directly into the stomach. Perhaps the most practical treatment is to feed liquid diets in an elevated position, eliminating the need for hard swallowing. The prognosis is *fair* to *guarded*

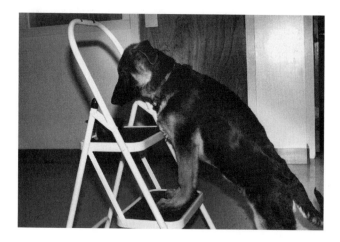

This dog is eating on a stool to help alleviate its megaesophagus. Because its head is higher than its stomach, the food (liquified) has a better chance of going down.

because these puppies don't thrive and are often stunted in growth. Breeders call these puppies "poor-doers."

Megaesophagus. This literally means "large esophagus." The esophagus is the tube that carries the swallowed food into the stomach. If the esophagus is dilated or enlarged, the food collects there and never makes it to the stomach. Factors that can cause a dilated esophagus are 1) impaired nerve control to the muscles of the esophagus as in a disease like myasthenia gravis (*see* page 37), so that the normal pushing along of the food (called peristalsis) stops; 2) genetic ballooning of the walls of the esophagus; and 3) reduced thyroid function. The breeds most often afflicted are the Great Dane and the German Shepherd Dog. The main symptom is that the puppy regurgitates within minutes to hours after eating solid foods. Regurgitation means the food just swallowed comes back up undigested (because it never made it to the stomach), without forceful stomach contractions (as seen in vomiting). Obviously, the puppy cannot get proper nutrition this way. Diagnosis is made when a history of regurgitation is established and an X ray is taken of the esophagus after having the puppy swallow a contrast medium (such as barium). The bloated esophagus is outlined by the contrast material and is easily seen. Treatment is simple: a fluid diet is fed, with the puppy's forequarters elevated to let gravity pull the food down into the stomach. Dry dog food is put into a blender with water to make a gruel or slurry, and the puppy is fed on a step stool. Many puppies outgrow this condition, so the prognosis is *fair*.

Pancreatic Insufficiency. This congenital condition exists when a puppy is born without sufficient alpha cells of the pancreas. These cells are responsible for secreting digestive enzymes needed for the proper digestion of fats, proteins and carbohydrates. The breeds most often seen with this condition are German Shepherd Dogs, setters, retrievers and most large breeds. If the digestive enzymes are lacking, the puppy cannot digest its food. Afflicted puppies are thin, undersized and have a poor growth rate. Their stools are soft, light-colored, continual, greasy and smelly. Their abdomens are bloated, and their owners complain of excess gas. Diagnosis is made with physical inspection of the stools and a laboratory test called a *fecal digestion study*, which demonstrates the undigested food components in the stool. It also checks for the presence of some digestive enzymes. Once the diagnosis is made, treatment can be started. An enzyme supplement is given with each meal. The diet should be a highly digestible food with low fiber and fat. The feedings should be small and frequent (three to four times daily).

These dogs cannot stray from their diet at all. Females seem more prone to this condition. Treatment is usually successful and must be continued for the puppy's life. The prognosis is *good*.

Persistent Right Aortic Arch. This is the most common of the congenital defects known as the *vascular ring anomalies*. The breeds most often seen with this condition are the German Shepherd Dog, Irish Setter and Boston Terrier. It has also been reported in the Labrador Retriever. You may be wondering why something to do with the heart and aorta is here under digestive disorders. I will explain.

The heart has several main blood vessels that carry blood toward and away from it. The main blood vessel that carries blood away from the heart and into the body is the *aorta*. A normal animal has only one aorta. A puppy with this defect, however, is born with two aortas: the left one, which is the large functional one that should be there, and a smaller right one that should have shriveled up and disappeared before birth. Therefore, the right aorta is called persistent. Why all the fuss about this remnant of a right aorta? Because the right aorta entraps the esophagus and constricts it (therein lies the term "vascular ring"). The result is a condition almost identical to that involving the megaesophagus, described previously in this section.

The symptoms are the same: chronic regurgitation of food. Diagnosis is also the same: a complete history of when the puppy regurgitates and a radiograph with contrast material to outline the distended esophagus. Treatment, however, is different. Surgery is needed to cut the persistent right aorta, freeing the strangulated esophagus. Wet slurry foods are also fed with the puppy in an elevated position (with its forequarters raised) for several weeks post-surgery to encourage easy transport of food into the stomach. Complications to the surgery include malnutrition and pneumonia (the puppy often aspirates the food into the lungs, where an infection starts). Sometimes the esophagus remains distended even after surgery. Either sex can be affected. Due to the necessity of surgery with its complications, the prognosis is *guarded*.

Ear Defects

Only two types of ear defects are commonly seen in weaned puppies. The first deals with the external ear and ear flap. The second deals with the inner ear and its nerve.

Cauliflower Ear. This is a catch-all phrase used to describe a variety of misshapen ear flaps. Usually only one side is affected. The ear flap can

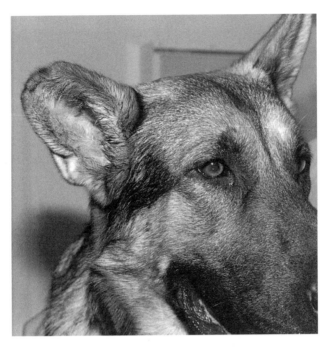

This misshapen ear is referred to as "cauliflower ear."

vary from being smaller, deformed in shape or even absent. Since this problem is primarily cosmetic, surgical treatment is needed only if appearance is important. There is no sex predilection. The prognosis is *good* to *excellent*.

Deafness. Deafness is a congenital condition predominantly of Dalmatians. The breeder or new owner notices that the puppy is not responding to sounds or voices. People can actually sneak up behind the puppy while it's sleeping and bang a pan or clap their hands in an attempt to startle the sleeping beauty. Deafness is due to a faulty inner ear, which is critical for transmitting sound from the environment to the nerve that picks up the sound and converts it into hearing in the brain. Sophisticated tests are available that can actually measure the amount of sound transmitted through the inner ear (called electroencephalography, or EEG). This test generally is not needed in veterinary medicine. Deaf puppies make great pets, but obviously some allowances have to be made for their hearing impairment. In fact, these dogs can be trained with hand signals instead of voice commands. The prognosis is *good*, as this condition is more of a handicap than a serious health concern.

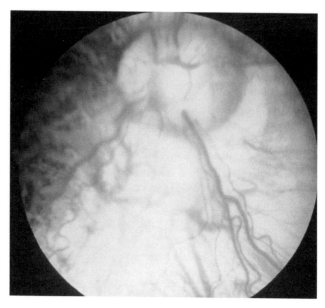

Collie eye, a defect noticed by eight weeks of age, is an ocular defect affecting mostly Collies and Shetland Sheepdogs. *Dr. M. Neaderland.*

Eye Defects

This category is the largest in this section. You'd be surprised how many things can go wrong in the development of the eyes. The following is an alphabetical list and description of the most common congenital eye defects that vets see around eight weeks of age.

> **Collie Eye.** As the name implies, this ocular defect occurs mainly in Collies, but Shetland Sheepdogs also are prone to it. As many as 80 percent of Collies may have the recessive gene for this defect. It is noticed by eight weeks of age. The retinas of these dogs are defective and immature (called *retinal dysplasia*) and have areas that are raised and pitted near the optic nerve (which are called *coloboma*). The eye itself is usually smaller than normal (which is called *microphthalmia*). All this translates into poor vision and blind spots. If the retina actually detaches, complete blindness will result, as seen in up to 4 percent of the cases. No treatment is available. Obviously, these dogs should not be bred. The only good thing about this condition is that it is not progressive. The prognosis is *guarded*, as many of these dogs are mostly blind.

> **Corneal Opacities.** These are white areas that cloud up the cornea (the clear surface of the eye). The cause can be either swelling of the

cornea or calcium deposits. They are most often seen in puppies born with their eyes open. No treatment is needed, and they spontaneously resolve. Breeds afflicted are the Doberman Pinscher, Toy Fox Terrier and Basenji. These opacities often are seen along with another condition known as persistent pupillary membrane, which is described later in this section. The prognosis is *good*.

Dermoids. A dermoid is a benign tumor of the tissues surrounding the eye, such as the conjunctiva or cornea. The tumor consists of tissue cells and hair follicles. There is often hair growing out of these, which can cause irritation to the eye. The dermoid of the cornea (the surface of the eye) blocks vision. The breeds that carry the gene for dermoid are the Pekingese, Poodle, Shih Tzu and Lhasa Apso. The only treatment for these growths is surgical removal. The only complication is post-surgical scarring, depending on how deep the dermoid was. The prognosis is *good* for the health of the dog and *fair* for its vision, depending on how much scarring results.

Distichiasis. This is an extra row of eyelashes that jut out of the upper or lower lid and rub against the cornea. The puppy has obvious signs of discomfort of the eye, such as excess tearing and squinting. The owners notice that one eye is always weeping and that the puppy keeps that eye partially closed as if something were always in it. The breeds most affected are the Poodles (miniature and toy varieties), Bulldog, Cocker Spaniel and Pekingese. The treatment is permanent removal of these extra lashes through electrolysis of each individual lash. If a corneal

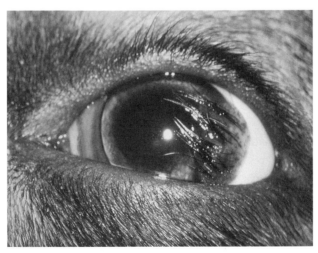

This dog has a dermoid, a benign tumor of the tissues surrounding the eye.
Dr. M. Neaderland

abrasion is also present, it is treated with triple antibiotic ophthalmic ointment three times daily. Either sex can be afflicted. The prognosis is *good* with treatment.

Ectropion. This condition is when the lower lid droops and everts outward. The look is of saggy, sad eyes. We see this most often in the hounds, Saint Bernard and Cocker Spaniel; it is a natural feature for these breeds and is considered normal. But excessive drooping of the lower lid can lead to chronic conjunctivitis and excessive tearing. Therefore, in extreme cases, it needs surgical correction. A variety of techniques are used, but most of them attempt to tuck the lower lid in order to eliminate some loose skin. The prognosis is *good*.

Entropion. This is the opposite of the ectropion condition just described. In entropion, either eyelid rolls inward so that the eyelashes actually rub against the cornea, causing corneal abrasions. Entropion is most common in the lower lid. Symptoms are corneal irritation (which includes excess tearing), squinting, redness of the sclera (the white of the eye), and a thick discharge. The breeds that have congenital entropion are the Labrador Retriever, Irish Setter, Bulldog, Saint Bernard, Newfoundland, Chow Chow, Great Dane and Chinese Shar Pei. Treatment is surgical correction. A slip of skin of the lid in question is removed, causing the lid to roll outward. Sometimes not enough tissue is removed during surgery, so the procedure must be redone. Some scarring is expected. The prognosis is *good*. If a corneal ulcer is present, this also must be treated with triple antibiotic ophthalmic ointment three times daily.

Iris Cysts. These are bizarre balloon-like structures that are attached to the iris of the eye. The iris is the colored aperture of the eye. It is the blue structure in blue eyes; the brown structure, in brown eyes. These fluid-filled sacs can break off and float around in the front chamber of the eye. No treatment exists. No breed or sex is prone to the condition. The cysts are mostly a nuisance, and the prognosis is *good*.

Juvenile Cataracts. A cataract is an opacity of the lens of the eye. If the opacity is greater than 50 percent, vision is diminished. Many factors contribute to cataract formation. Age and diabetes mellitus are certainly two of the most well-known. But this discussion is restricted to cataracts of puppies less than six months old. Juvenile cataracts are inherited in several hound breeds, the Cocker Spaniel, German Shepherd Dog, retrievers, Poodle, Miniature Schnauzer and others. Perhaps the Golden Retriever is the most prone. They can be in either one eye (unilateral) or both (bilateral). Some of the cataracts mature, or get more opaque; others are not progressive and stay immature (or small—that's good!). Diagnosis is made on physical exam with a slit-lamp ophthalmoscope. Treatment is only for the very thick, pearl-like, opaque lenses that block vision. The cloudy lens must be removed surgically by a qualified veterinary ophthalmologist. Prior to surgery, the health of the retina must be

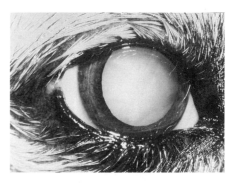

Cataracts, opacities of the lens of the eye, are usually a problem of old age, but puppies can get them, too. *Dr. M. Neaderland*

evaluated to ensure that vision will be restored once the defective lens is removed. This is done by an electroretinogram (ERG). The prognosis is *fair* to *good* depending on the severity of the cataract and the success of the surgery. Complications are common after this surgery.

Night Blindness. This is a defect or deficiency of those areas of the retina (namely, the rods) that are needed to see in low-light situations. Owners or breeders complain that the puppy sees fine during the day, but at dusk and at night he starts to walk into things. A definitive diagnosis is made by a veterinary ophthalmologist. The two breeds this is seen in are the Tibetan Terrier and the Briard. This is one form of retinal dysplasia, which is described at the end of this section. No treatment exists, but since the puppies are only affected at night, the prognosis is usually *good.*

Persistent Pupillary Membrane (PPM). During the fetal development of the eye, a thin membrane covers the pupil area. At birth this membrane is supposed to disintegrate, leaving the pupillary aperture open in the center of the eye. Occasionally, this membrane leaves strings or cobweb-like strands that span across the pupil. As mentioned earlier under "Corneal Opacities," these strands can cause cloudiness of the cornea wherever they touch it. This condition is hereditary in the Basenji, but we see it often in other breeds. There is no treatment, and PPMs only affect the vision if they cause severe corneal opacity. The prognosis is *good.*

Retinal Dysplasia. This term refers to a collection of congenital defects of the retina. The retina is the inner lining of the back of the eye that receives the light that comes through the lens and converts it to

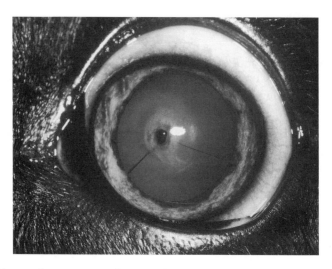

When a thin membrane covering the eye fails to disintegrate at birth, it leaves the pupillary aperture open in the center of the eye, a condition called persistent pupillary membrane. *Dr. M. Neaderland.*

nerve impulses to the brain. (The optic nerve stems from the retina at the optic disc.) Therefore, retinal function is essential for proper vision. A mild form of retinal dysplasia was already described under "Night Blindness." The sporting breeds seem to have more of this defect than others, especially the Labrador Retriever and the Cocker Spaniel. Other breeds that have been noted are the Beagle, Bedlington Terrier, Sealyham Terrier and Springer Spaniel. Symptoms start as young as six to eight weeks of age. The puppies start by having difficulty seeing at night, then start having trouble seeing during the day. Owners say that the puppies can't see a ball or stick thrown to them. Clearly these dogs should not be used for breeding. No treatment exists, and the prognosis is *guarded* to *poor* for vision.

Heart Defects

Unfortunately, puppies are sometimes born with heart defects. These do not manifest themselves until about eight weeks of age or older. The ones listed here are those that usually show up early. The veterinarian is the one to detect these defects at the first physical exam. Listening to the heart with a stethoscope enables the vet to hear certain sounds characteristic of these defects, such as heart murmurs. Most of these defects are serious and require surgical correction. These are the three most common:

Aortic Stenosis. This congenital defect is the third-most-common one seen in puppies. Stenosis means "narrowing." In these cases the aortic valves (the valves are the doors that open and allow blood to flow through) are narrowed to the point of almost constricting the outflow of blood from the aorta. The aorta is the main artery that carries blood away from the heart and supplies oxygenated blood to the entire body. You can imagine the trouble caused by cutting this flow by as much as half! Early symptoms include trouble breathing, loss of energy, coughing and paleness of the mucous membranes of the mouth. In other words, symptoms of *congestive heart failure*. The first thing the veterinarian hears is a loud murmur on the left side of the chest, which radiates up to the throat. The heart rate is too fast (called *tachycardia*), and the pulse is weak.

Diagnostic tests could include chest X rays, electrocardiograms and ultrasound. Of the three, the ultrasound (called an *echocardiogram*) is the most helpful. Radiographs using contrast material to highlight the narrowed aorta (called *angiography*) are also helpful in visualizing the stenosis. The breeds most often affected are the Newfoundland, Golden Retriever, Boxer and German Shepherd Dog. Other breeds have also been diagnosed, including the Bulldog and Basset Hound. The treatment is open-chest surgical correction of the stenosis. Depending on the extent of the narrowing, the prognosis is *guarded* to *poor*. A substantial percentage of these puppies die suddenly of cardiac arrhythmia.

Pulmonic Stenosis. As described in "Aortic Stenosis," stenosis refers to the narrowing of the outflow valves of the blood vessel—in this case, the pulmonic artery. This artery is the main vessel that carries unoxygenated blood to the lungs. This is the second-most-common congenital heart defect of puppies. Affected breeds are Beagles, Samoyeds, Miniature Schnauzers and Chihuahuas. Constriction causes a backup of blood pressure in the right side of the heart, causing a right-sided heart failure.

Symptoms include trouble breathing, weakness and fainting. These signs can be mild at a young age and worsen with time. The first thing a veterinarian notices is a heart murmur on the left side. Electrocardiograms and X rays of the chest are usually normal. In severe cases, these tests will show enlargement of the right side of the heart. Echocardiography (the use of ultrasound to visualize the heart muscle in motion) is the best tool to diagnose this condition. Angiography, or the use of contrast material to outline the dilated blood vessel on X ray, is also helpful. Without treatment, these dogs live into early adulthood only. Surgery is the only corrective option. Without surgery, the prognosis is *poor*; with surgery, it is *fair*.

Patent Ductus Arteriosus (PDA). This is the number-one congenital heart defect of dogs. Veterinarians see it in the Pomeranian, Collie, Shetland Sheepdog, Miniature Poodle and German Shepherd. The following explanation is a little complicated, but try to stay with me. During the development of the fetus, a duct exists between the left pulmonary artery and the aorta. This causes the blood to bypass the lungs because the lungs are not functional in the fetus. At birth, this channel closes, directing the newborn's blood to the lungs so that it can breathe air. If the arterial duct (or *ductus arteriosus*) remains open (patent), then there is a shunting of blood through the duct from the aorta to the pulmonary artery. This overloads the artery and floods the lungs with blood. The consequences are wet lungs, difficulty breathing, rapid respiratory rate and, eventually, death.

The veterinarian hears a very loud murmur on the left side of the chest wall. The left side of the heart is stressed from the increased pressure in the lungs and enlarges to compensate. The aorta can even develop a bulge from the pressure (called an *aneurysm*). Diagnosis is made by an electrocardiogram and chest X ray, which show left-sided heart enlargement. Angiography with contrast material to demonstrate the duct confirms the diagnosis. Treatment is always surgical ligation (tying off) of the duct. Since this is open thoracic surgery, it should be performed by a qualified veterinary surgeon. The prognosis is *fair* to *good* with surgery.

Ventricular Septal Defect (VSD). This defect is a hole in the wall (or *septa*) between the left and right ventricles. This is a congenital "hole in the heart." Because the pressure is higher in the left ventricle than in the right, blood shunts from the left ventricle to the right one. All breeds can get this defect, but the Bulldog is especially prone. The signs are heart failure, coughing, loss of energy, pale mucous membranes, and a loud heart murmur that the veterinarian hears on the right side of the chest. Since electrocardiograms and chest X rays are generally normal, an echocardiogram (ultrasound of the heart) is the test of choice. The hole in the septa between the ventricles is easily visualized. Treatment is not required if the hole is small, but most dogs need to have the hole surgically closed. A graft or patch is used if the hole is too large to suture closed. This is open-heart surgery and should only be attempted by a board-certified veterinary surgeon. There are several postoperative complications, which warrant a *guarded* prognosis.

Hormonal Defects

Hormones are chemicals secreted by glands in the body that circulate in the blood to a specific organ, where they regulate and control certain bodily functions. For example, the ovaries of the female secrete the estrogen hormone, which targets the uterus and regulates the heat cycles in the bitch. Another example would be the thyroid gland, which secretes the thyroid hormone that regulates the body's metabolism and the rate at which food energy gets burned up. Since these hormones control crucial bodily functions, it is easy to see that if there were a defect in them, the consequences could be serious. The following are the most common hormonal defects seen in weanling puppies.

Hypoglycemia. Hypoglycemia literally means low blood sugar. Most of us think of this when we've gone all day without eating and we start to get tired. This is a very mild and temporary form of hypoglycemia. Think how you would feel if you had dangerously low levels of blood sugar all the time. This is what we see in certain puppies. The mechanism for regulating blood sugar levels is very complex and beyond the scope of this chapter. Suffice it to say that hormones are needed in this process. Glucagon and insulin are the main ones that control blood sugar levels. Insulin lowers blood sugar levels and is discussed later in this section. Glucagon raises blood sugar levels and is needed to mobilize sugars stored in the fat and liver when there isn't enough coming from food sources. This mobilization brings the blood glucose (the sugar of blood) up to normal levels. There needs to be balance between insulin and glucagon.

It is important that the liver be healthy because glucose mobilization occurs in that organ. Other hormones are involved, such as adrenaline and cortisol, which help raise the glucose level. The most common cause of hypoglycemia in neonates is food deprivation. If the puppy goes too long without eating, or is lactose-intolerant and cannot digest the milk, then blood glucose levels drop. Also, if there is a deficiency of glucagon, adrenaline or cortisol hormones, the same will happen. These puppies are weak, underdeveloped, motionless unless coaxed, and mentally dull and disoriented. They can even have seizures. Some die within several weeks of whelping. The diagnosis is made by checking blood glucose level. Normally, the level should be between 60 and 140mg/dl. But in these puppies, it is below 40mg/dl. In all cases, the liver function should be tested. Treatment of mild hypoglycemia is with oral glucose or other sugar supplements. Owners will also have to ensure that the puppy gets regular feedings so as not to allow the blood glucose levels to fall too low. The severe cases of disorientation, collapse or seizures require veterinary treatment of intravenous fluids rich in glucose or other easily metabolized sugars. The severe cases carry a *guarded* to *poor* prognosis because this problem does not correct itself with age. There is no breed or sex predilection for this defect.

Juvenile Diabetes mellitus. This is the most common hormonal disorder of puppies. In these dogs, a high level of blood glucose (sugar) is present all the time, not just after feedings. In people, juvenile diabetes is insulin *dependent*, meaning that insulin levels are low. Adult-onset diabetes is insulin *non-dependent*, which means that the body has normal levels of insulin but the tissues do not recognize or utilize it. Insulin is secreted by the beta cells in the Islets of Langerhans region of the pancreas. Diabetes mellitus is characterized by consistently high levels of glucose in the blood and urine (as blood sugar levels rise above 200mg/dl, it overflows into the urine via the kidneys). Normal levels of blood glucose fall in the 60-to-140mg/dl range.

Symptoms include increased thirst and, therefore, increased urine output; cataract development in the eyes; loss of energy and weight (even though the blood has an abundance of glucose, without insulin the body can't use it, and these dogs are actually starving); poor circulation; and, often, concurrent heart disease. As you can see, this disease is very serious. Factors that increase the chances of diabetes are obesity and poor breeding. Estrogen, which is the female hormone in unspayed bitches, also seems to be involved in decreasing the effects of insulin. Therefore, diabetes mellitus may be a complex of hormonal imbalances in the female.

Because diabetes in animals is usually due to a lack of insulin, the treatment is to give insulin injections daily. This must be done under close supervision of a veterinarian. The correct dose must be tailored to the individual. The owner is told to check the level of glucose in the urine each morning, using a color-coded stick (available at any pharmacy) held under the morning urine stream. The color changes relative to the amount of glucose in the urine: The darker the strip, the more glucose present. This check is done prior to the insulin injection so that the amount of insulin can be increased or decreased from the day before. Most veterinarians have a chart to use as a guide to figure out how much to increase or decrease the insulin based on the color of the urine glucose stick. Please remember, the blood glucose level changes dramatically during a given day and from day to day, so it must be monitored a minimum of once daily.

The vet aims at keeping the blood glucose level between 100 to 200mg/dl. The timing of feedings in relation to the injection is crucial to a successful treatment protocol. If the NPH form of insulin is used (it is the most common form for animals), then owners are instructed to feed the puppy immediately following the insulin shot, and again eight hours later, as this insulin has two peak actions eight hours apart.

The reason feedings are coordinated with the insulin shot is because as the insulin starts to work, it pulls down the blood sugar level. But as the food is digested, it raises the blood sugar level. Therefore, the level never goes too low (below 60mg/dl), as this would cause what's known as *insulin shock*. Insulin shock is when the effects of insulin pull the blood glucose level *too low*, and the animal suffers from hypoglycemia (discussed earlier). The treatment for this shock is to raise the blood glucose level quickly by smearing a super-sweet syrup in the mouth and gums, where it is instantly absorbed. Pancake syrup can be substituted in a pinch. The breeds most affected with juvenile diabetes are Golden and Labrador Retrievers, Old English Sheepdogs, Alaskan Malamutes, Keeshonds, Miniature Schnauzers, German Shepherd Dogs and Chow Chows. There is no sex predilection. With proper insulin management, most diabetics lead a normal life and the prog-nosis is *fair* to *good*.

Liver Defects

Young puppies are sometimes born with congenital defects of the liver. These range from mild to very serious. The following is an alphabetical listing of the most common liver defects seen in young puppies.

Copper Storage Disease of Bedlington and West Highland White Terriers. Two breeds have a recessive trait that causes a dangerously high accumulation of copper in the liver. As many as 66 percent of Bedlington Terriers have this recessive gene. Although there are often no symptoms at eight weeks of age, the copper starts accumulating at this time, and the liver starts being affected. Therefore, this defect is included in this section. Copper is a metal found in trace amounts in many foods. Copper is needed for strong bones and blood. In excess, copper is toxic to the liver. A normal liver maintains a certain level of copper. In afflicted dogs, the regulatory mechanism is faulty, resulting in too much copper stored in the liver. These toxic levels cause destruction of the liver cells, which leads to hepatitis (inflammation of the liver). Chronic hepatitis leads to scarring, or cirrhosis of the liver. This in turn leads to liver failure. The symptoms of liver failure are a yellowing of the mucous membranes (called *jaundice*), loss of appetite, vomiting, lethargy and weight loss.

Diagnosis is made with blood tests of the liver function. These include a chemistry screen of liver enzymes, serum copper levels, an ultrasound of the liver, bile acid tests for liver function and, ultimately, a liver biopsy. The treatment of this disease is with drugs named *penicillamine* or *trientine*. These drugs bind to the copper (called *chelating*) and lower the levels. Penicillamine can cause stomach upset, so it should be given with food. The liver does not regenerate itself, so whatever damage was done prior to treatment is permanent. All foods high in copper should be avoided, such as liver, shellfish, vitamin/mineral supplements that contain copper, and certain commercial dog foods. With treatment, most of these dogs do well, so the prognosis is *fair* to *good*.

Glycogen Storage Disease. Glycogen is an energy source that is stored in the liver and used when there is no food to utilize. Glycogen is used before fat during times of fasting. Glycogen storage disease results when glycogen cannot be mobilized out of the liver due to an enzyme deficiency. This means that if the dog goes too long without eating, its blood sugar starts to fall, and if glycogen cannot be released from the liver, the puppy becomes hypoglycemic (low blood sugar).

Symptoms are weakness, tremors and body shaking, depression and, occasionally, seizures. The glycogen continues to accumulate in the liver, causing that organ to enlarge. The veterinarian can palpate (feel) the enlarged liver and visualize it with either an X ray or ultrasound. A liver biopsy will demonstrate the glycogen buildup. Puppies start showing these symptoms between meals, as young as eight weeks of age. Frequent small feedings are needed to alleviate the symptoms. Since there are several different types of this condition, it is hard to generalize on a prognosis. In general, it is *guarded* to *fair*.

Portosystemic Shunts (PSS). This is the most common liver defect seen in young puppies. It is very complicated, so I may run the risk of oversimplifying, but try to follow along. In the normal puppy, the venous blood circulation from the intestines, which carries most of the nutritional products of digestion, flows through the liver via the portal veins. This is crucial for the liver to metabolize the digestive by-products. In puppies with portosystemic shunting, much of this intestinal venous blood bypasses the liver by another route, usually a vein other than the portal ones. This means that the blood carrying the digestive materials never gets metabolized through the liver. The consequences are dramatic.

These puppies are sickly from birth, but by eight weeks show stunted growth, persistent vomiting and diarrhea, weight loss, drug reactions and neurologic symptoms, including strange behavior and seizures (called *hepatic encephalopathy*). Blood sugar and protein levels are usually low, and ammonia levels are dangerously high. All these are worsened by a large high-protein meal, because the venous blood from the intestines, which carries the proteins, sugars, ammonia and waste products, never gets processed in the liver. Blood serum chemistry tests show liver enzyme increases. The bile acid blood test shows grossly elevated levels, proving the liver deficiency.

The livers of these puppies are much smaller than normal, as seen on X ray. Liver biopsy reveals changes indicative of liver dysfunction. The shunting of venous blood can be visualized with either ultrasound or contrast X rays (called *portovenography*), which highlight the shunting blood around the liver. These shunting veins can be either inside or outside the liver itself.

Treatment is surgical ligation (tying-off) of the shunting veins in order to divert the intestinal blood flow back through the liver. Obviously, those shunts outside the liver are easier to get to. The surgery is very tricky and should be done only by a qualified veterinary surgeon. Sudden tying off of the shunting vein can cause a rapid increase of pressure to the liver, causing hypertension. The surgeon must be careful not to tie it off too quickly so that the liver has a chance to acclimate to the higher pressure. Puppies that survive the surgery need to be on a protein-restricted diet for the rest of their lives. Some experts believe that antibiotics, which limit the amount of ammonia produced by digestive bacteria, help. There are even medications that lower blood ammonia levels. There is no breed or sex predilection. Due to the serious nature of this condition, the prognosis is *guarded* to *poor*.

Neurological Defects

By the time puppies are eight weeks old, you can begin to appreciate how mobile they are, like a one-year-old baby. Nothing is better than seeing a litter of eight-week-old puppies running around, frolicking and playing. It becomes painfully obvious when one is left out due to lack of coordination. Most owners notice quickly when one is doing strange things like head pressing, circling, falling to one side, flickering its eyes and so on. Defects of the neurologic system can start in the brain, spinal cord, or nervous network.

I have already touched on some neurological problems secondary to other defects, like hepatic encephalopathy (under "Portosystemic Shunts (PSS)" in the "Liver Defects" section), and "Hydrocephalus" (under "Skeletal Defects"). The following defects are primary neurological ones; that is, the defect is in the nervous system itself.

Cerebellar Hypoplasia. This literally means that the cerebellum section of the brain is underdeveloped and small-sized. The cerebellum is the part of the brain that controls coordination and regulates body movement. This defect is inherited in certain breeds, such as the Irish Setter, Fox Terrier and Chow Chow. Clinically, these puppies can barely walk, or they have grossly exaggerated motions. They shake, jerk and have head tremors. Some people find this cute at first, but it quickly becomes obvious that there is something terribly wrong. These cases vary from slightly affected to seriously disabled. The mild cases can go undiagnosed for months. By this age, the symptoms stabilize and are nonprogressive.

No treatment exists for either the progressive or nonprogressive forms. Severe cases may need to be euthanized, but the mild cases can make wonderful pets. These dogs cannot be used for work or sporting purposes that require good balance and coordination. It should also be noted that puppies born perfectly healthy can develop cerebellar symptoms from an infection of the distemper virus. The prognosis for the mild cases is *guarded*, whereas for the severe or progressive cases it is *poor*.

Narcolepsy. This condition is an odd one. A defect in the brain stem causes the dog to sleep uncontrollably, so these puppies literally fall asleep while playing or eating. The brain stem defect causes inappropriate rapid-eye-movement sleep patterns. At first the owner thinks the puppy is simply tired; it soon becomes obvious there is something wrong when he falls asleep in his feed bowl. The puppy may slumber thirty, forty or more times daily for several minutes each time. The dogs may actually have their eyes open while sleeping, so "sleep" may not be the correct term. Stirring them can bring them out of it sooner. Luckily, the symptoms tend to lessen with age. The breeds most affected are the Labrador Retriever and Doberman Pinscher. Diagnosis is made by observing the puppy during these "sleep attacks." Treatment is not very effective but consists of trying not to get the puppy too excited, as this can start the sleep cycle. Antidepressant drugs may help.

The prognosis is *fair*, but these dogs can never make completely normal pets.

Vestibular Disorders. The word *vestibular* refers to the inner ear. The inner ear is needed to maintain balance, normal head position and equilibrium. A puppy that loses its balance or equilibrium, tilts its head, and walks in circles or falls over to one side is exhibiting classic symptoms of a vestibular problem. The breed most affected is the German Shepherd Dog. These symptoms are in full effect by eight weeks of age. Many puppies grow out of this condition and compensate, although a persistent head tilt is common. No treatment is available, and the prognosis is *guarded* to *fair*.

Respiratory Defects

This group of defects involves the respiratory tract. The respiratory tract is divided into two areas: the upper respiratory tract, which includes the nose, nostrils, sinuses, throat, larynx (Adam's apple) and part of the trachea (windpipe); and the lower respiratory tract, which includes the lower trachea, major and minor bronchial tubes and the lungs themselves. You will note that the defects are classified as affecting either the upper or lower tract.

Collapsing Trachea. Think of the trachea (or windpipe) as being like a vacuum cleaner hose, made up of rings so that it's flexible. These rings keep the hose open and round. If rings are missing or broken, then the hose is weak in those spots and collapses or flattens slightly under pressure. The trachea of affected puppies is like a defective vacuum cleaner hose: They are born with defective or missing cartilage rings of the trachea. The defect can occur anywhere along the trachea, either in the throat or inside the chest. This is the only respiratory defect that can affect both the upper and lower tract.

This weakness causes the trachea to collapse slightly when the puppy is breathing heavily. This sets off a coughing spasm that sounds like a goose-honking, which lasts until the puppy calms down and catches its breath. The breeds most often affected are the brachycephalic breeds (the ones with pushed-in faces) like the Pekingese, Bulldog and Boston Terrier, and the toy breeds such as the Chihuahua, Yorkshire Terrier, Toy Poodle and Pomeranian. A few other breeds have been noted as well, such as the Chinese Shar-Pei.

Diagnosis is made after a history of coughing or "goose-honking" on exertion has been established, and tests are performed, including a physical exam, an X ray that shows the area of collapse, or an endoscopic exam where the vet can actually visualize the affected stretch of trachea. The medical treatment available is limited. The puppy should be kept from doing strenuous exercise, kept thin so that fat doesn't put additional pressure on the throat, and be given cough suppressants. Other than in surgical cases, the prognosis is *fair*.

Diaphragmatic Hernia. You may be wondering why this defect is included here with the respiratory defects. The reason is that the diaphragm is the main muscle involved in breathing. This thin sheet-like muscle separates the chest cavity from the abdomen. It contracts with every breath. If this muscle had a tear or opening in it, the stomach, liver and small intestines would pass through into the chest! Some puppies are born with such a tear or gap in the diaphragm. Vets are not sure whether a genetic basis exists for this defect or whether it happens during the strong contractions of whelping. By eight weeks of age, certain symptoms are noticeable, such as labored breathing, lack of endurance, weight loss, and digestive disorders. German Shepherd Dogs seem to be the breed most commonly affected, with males and females having equal incidence. A veterinarian is needed to make the diagnosis. The vet can clearly hear with a stethoscope the gut sounds in the chest, and the heart sounds are usually muffled. An X ray of the chest clearly shows loops of bowel or stomach in the chest. Treatment is always surgical. Basically, the hole needs to be closed. The anesthesia is very tricky with this surgery due to the lack of integrity of the chest wall. These dogs require respiratory assistance during surgery. Closure of a hernia is called *herniorrhaphy*. The difficulty of the surgery is related to the size of the hernia. Therefore, the larger the hernia, the poorer the prognosis. Scarring and break down of the repair area are common complications. Technically, this is neither an upper nor lower respiratory disease. Generally, the prognosis is *guarded*.

Emphysema. Most of us think of this as a disease of older people who smoke. But vets see it in young puppies, too. *Emphysema* refers to the trapping of air in the lung tissues. You may say, "What's wrong with air in the lung tissues? Isn't that where it's supposed to be?" Well, yes, but the function of the lungs is to exchange oxygen and carbon dioxide between the air and blood. This necessitates that air flow in and out of the lung tissues freely. The oxygen from the air saturates the blood in the pulmonary capillaries of the lung tissue so as to oxygenate the blood (make it oxygen rich). The wasteproduct carbon dioxide comes from the venous blood to the lungs, where it is transferred to the lung tissue so that it can be exhaled out of the body with the next breath. You can imagine that anything which inhibits the flow of air in and out of the lungs affects these gas exchanges and, therefore, respiration. In emphysema, the lung tissues are dilated, so air is trapped and cannot flow out easily. These puppies have trouble pushing air *out* of their lungs; they labor to breathe, have no exercise tolerance, and turn blue (cyanotic) upon the slightest exertion. With a stethoscope, the veterinarian can hear crackles, harsh lung sounds and wheezes. X rays of the chest show areas of trapped air in distended lung tissue. No treatment for this defect exists other than having the puppy avoid stress or exertion. Since the lungs are involved, this is a lower respiratory disease. There is no breed or sex predilection. The prognosis is generally *poor*.

Stenotic Nares. This literally translates to "narrowed nostrils." This is strictly an upper respiratory defect. Certain breeds like the Pug, Pekingese, Boston Terrier, Bulldog and Shih Tzu are most affected. Their nostrils are narrow, constricting air flow. Some cases are so severe that the puppy cannot breathe through its nose at all! These puppies are open-mouth breathers. They also make a lot of snorting and snuffling noises when they breathe. Mild cases do not need any treatment; more severe cases need surgical correction of the nostrils. A wedge of the cartilage in the nose is removed, permanently opening it up. This is the canine equivalent of a nose job. The prognosis is *good* in all cases.

Miscellaneous Defects Noticed at Eight Weeks of Age
Trick Knees

The other name for this condition is *medial* or *lateral luxating patella*. Medial means "toward the inside," and lateral means "toward the outside." The medial luxating patella means that the patella, or kneecap, luxates (pops out of joint) toward the inside of the leg. The lateral luxating patella means the kneecap pops out toward the outside of the leg. Toy breeds commonly get the medial version, whereas large breeds get the lateral type. In either case, what happens is that the groove in which the patella sits is too shallow. This allows the patella to pop out of joint when the knee joint is flexed. Trick knees are graded from I to IV in severity: Grade I means you have to try manually to dislocate the kneecap. Grade IV is when the patella is permanently out of joint.

Symptoms include short bouts of lameness on the hind leg when the kneecap pops out and then back into joint. On palpation of the stifle, the vet can feel that the kneecap is obviously not in its groove. The veterinarian should always check the kneecaps in puppies of this age group as part of a physical exam. An X ray is also useful for visualizing the popped-out knee-cap. If symptoms are mild and infrequent, no treatment is needed. In more severe cases, surgery is needed to correct the defect. Several techniques have been developed to rebuild the ligaments that hold the kneecap in place, along with deepening the groove in the trochlea of the femur. An ortho-pedic veterinary surgeon is often required. The prognosis in mild cases with-out surgery, as well as in the more severe cases with surgery, is *good*.

Undescended Testicles

This is a condition know by most breeders as *cryptorchidism*. In this defect, one of the testicles in the male usually doesn't descend into the scrotum shortly after birth, as it normally should. That testicle is considered "retained," meaning it stayed in the abdomen. The defect is an autosomal recessive ge-netic trait, with the incidence of right-sided retention being twice that of the left side. The overall incidence is about 1 percent. Although the text-books say that after two months if the testicle hasn't descended, it won't, I have seen testicles drop in the third or fourth month of age. By the time the puppy is five months old, the chances of it dropping are slim to none. Occasionally the testicle gets stuck in the inguinal region (the opening the testicle would normally go through). This is still classified as an unde-scended testicle. At one time it was fashionable to use a human hormone called *human chorionic gonadotropin* to treat these cases, but science has proved that it does not help. The only treatment for this is to surgically remove the testicles or castrate the dog when it is of age, usually around six months. The reason for castration is twofold. First, this is a genetic flaw and should not be propagated by breeding. Second, the retained testicle is more prone to twisting and developing cancer. Therefore, castration is indicated as a preventive measure.

Defects Noticed by Six Months of Age

The congenital and inherited defects described in this section are not gener-ally seen before six months of age. Therefore, it is important to have your puppy rechecked at this age, since these puppies have been placed into their new homes and are quickly becoming new members of the family. This age is also the time most owners spay or neuter their dog. This is a wonderful op-portunity for the veterinarian to check for these problems before surgery. As in the other sections, the defects are listed under headings when there is more than one in the group, and they are listed alphabetically.

Blood Abnormalities

There are too many blood defects to list in this book, and most of them are very rare and affect only one breed—for example, cyclic hematopoiesis of the silver-gray Collie, or anemia of Alaskan Malamutes and Miniature Poodles. Therefore, this section lists the most common disorders that affect many breeds. These blood aberrations rarely show up before the puppy is two months old and may not show up until six months.

Autoimmune Hemolytic Anemia (AIHA). This is an odd condition in which the puppy's immune system actually seeks out and destroys its own red blood cells, resulting in an anemia. An *anemia* is defined as a reduction of red blood cells in the blood below normal levels (normally, blood should be between 37 to 52 percent red blood cells to transport oxygen effectively to the body's tissues). Why this happens is still a mystery, but it does. Perhaps there is a viral component, because anemia often follows viral infections. These anemias are classified as "regenerative," which means that the bone marrow of the puppy replaces the destroyed red blood cells with new ones. Unfortunately, the new ones are not as useful as the older destroyed ones, because they are immature and carry less oxygen. The puppy suffers from poor oxygenation of its tissues.

Symptoms include pale mucous membranes of the mouth, lack of energy (lethargy), amber discoloration of the urine, and a severely reduced red blood cell count. The disorder is diagnosed with physical findings on exam, and blood tests that include a complete blood count (CBC) and a Coombs test. Treatment is aggressive, with use of fairly high doses of corticosteroids, iron supplements, blood transfusions as needed and possibly a splenectomy (surgical removal of the spleen because this organ plays a role in the destruction of the red blood cells). The prognosis is variable. If the puppy responds initially to the treatment, then it is *fair*. If there is little response, the prognosis worsens to *poor*.

Aplastic Anemia. Fortunately, this congenital defect is not too common. Unlike the AIHA just described, this anemia isn't regenerative (it's non-regenerative). And it's not just the red blood cells that are reduced; it's also the white blood cells and the platelet cells, which are used in forming blood clots. This is due to a suppression of the bone marrow, where these blood cells are made. These poor puppies don't just have poorly oxygenated tissues, they also have a malfunctioning immune system (thanks to the reduced white blood cells) and a coagulopathy (poor clotting of the blood because of reduced platelet cells). As you can imagine, these are very sick puppies. The diagnosis is the same as for AIHA just described, but with a bone marrow biopsy as well. Treatment also involves heavy doses of corticosteroids, iron supplements and blood transfusions as needed. The splenectomy is not indicated, because in this condition it is not a matter of the blood cells being destroyed; they are not being manufactured by the bone marrow in the first place. Drugs used to stimulate the bone marrow are also used. The prognosis is *guarded* to *poor*.

Polycythemia. Polycythemia literally means too many red blood cells. This is the opposite of anemia. Polycythemic blood actually becomes muddy in consistency. Three types of this condition exist: 1. *Relative polycythemia* is due to excess fluid loss from the blood volume, usually from severe dehydration. 2. *Absolute polycythemia* is when the bone marrow pumps out far too many red blood cells because the bone marrow is over-stimulated by the *erythropoietin* hormone, which regulates red blood cell production. The body naturally produces this hormone as a response to situations that stress the body's red blood cells, such as high altitudes, poor circulation, and certain diseases. The cause is unknown, and the condition is rare. 3. *Secondary polycythemia* is the third type and means that it is secondary to another problem, the most common being congenital heart defects with blood shunting, and kidney or ovarian tumors. The diagnosis of all three types is made using the complete blood count blood test, where the percentage of the red blood cells in the blood consistently exceeds 70 percent. Also, the mucous membranes of the mouth are dry and ruddy in color. The condition is managed with certain drugs, such as hydroxyurea, which slows down the production of red blood cells. Prognosis is *fair* for these puppies.

Thrombocytopenia. This literally translates to "a decreased number of thrombocytes." What is a *thrombocyte*? This is a type of blood cell that is essential in forming a blood clot. Another name for a thrombocyte is a *platelet*. When bleeding occurs anywhere in the body, platelets are called upon to come together and form a clot. Obviously, when not enough platelets are circulating, it takes longer to form a clot. This delay in clotting time is called a *coagulopathy*. There are genetic causes of this deficiency in dogs. The defect seems to be in the bone marrow, where the platelets are manufactured. An autoimmune disorder has been observed. Certain drugs (like estrogen) and infectious diseases have also been known to cause thrombocytopenia. Collies seem to be prone to this. Symptoms are excessive bruising, prolonged bleeding from minor cuts or scratches, frequent nosebleeds, and bloody urine. Diagnosis is made with the clinical history, a low platelet count on a CBC test, and, in autoimmune cases, a Platelet Factor-3 test (this tests for antibodies against platelets). Treatment consists of avoiding cuts and abrasions, a blood transfusion if the platelet count gets below 20,000, a splenectomy (surgical removal of the spleen because it can destroy platelets), and cortisone drugs if an autoimmune factor is involved. The prognosis is *guarded*.

Von Willebrand's Disease (VWD). This is an inherited hemophilia of dogs. *Hemophilia* is defined as a lack of one of eight different coagulation factors. The factor missing in this case is Factor VIII. Coagulation factors are proteins that are crucial in the blood-clotting process. Without all eight of them, the blood clotting is severely delayed. This is true for people as well. This disorder is inherited, where males are affected and females are carriers. The breed most affected is the Doberman Pinscher, although it can occur in most breeds, especially the German Shepherd Dog, Golden Retriever, Schnauzer and Scottish Terrier. Symptoms are excessive bleeding, frequent nosebleeds, pale mucous membranes, easy bruising, and bloody urine. Owners notice that small abrasions or minor surgical procedures like tail docking bleed for up to an hour. Diagnosis is made with a coagulation blood test and a von Willebrand's test. The coagulation test determines the time it takes for a clot to form, whereas the von Willebrand's test actually measures the level of Factor VIII. Treatment is needed when the dog is in danger of hemorrhaging and usually means a whole-blood or plasma transfusion. Some veterinarians treat VWD with injections of vitamin K_1, as this vitamin aids in making the coagulation factors. I have also found it helpful. The prognosis is *guarded*.

Dental Defects

Dental defects of younger puppies were described in the previous section. There is one that doesn't show up until six months of age. It is described in this section. But first, let's look at what you should normally see in your puppy's mouth. The number and type of teeth normally found in any animal is called the *dental formula*. In dogs, this means there should be the following number and type of teeth:

An eight-week-old puppy should have, *on both sides of its mouth*, three upper and lower incisors, one upper and lower canine, and three upper and lower premolars.

A six-month-old puppy should have its permanent teeth and, *on both sides of its mouth*, three upper and lower incisors, one upper and lower canine, four upper and lower premolars, and two upper and three lower molars.

Teething. The stage when teeth cut through the gum line is called *teething*. Most puppies start cutting their deciduous (or puppy) teeth at six weeks of age. These puppy teeth suffice for a couple of months. When the puppy is four months old, the permanent teeth start erupting. The following table summarizes the timing of the permanent teeth:

Permanent Tooth Eruption	
Tooth Type	Eruption Time
Incisor	4 months
Canine	5 months
Premolar	6 months
Molars	6 to 7 months

Retained Deciduous Teeth. This is the most common defect of dentition of this age group. In this condition, a deciduous, or puppy tooth, doesn't fall out by six months of age. This has an impact two ways. First, it means an extra tooth will still be in place when the permanent tooth starts coming in. Second, the retained tooth may inhibit the permanent tooth from coming in, or coming in normally. In fact, the retained puppy tooth can cause the adult tooth to come in skewed. This condition is seen most often in toy breeds. Treatment is to remove the retained puppy tooth if it hasn't fallen out on its own by six months. We have removed them earlier if the permanent tooth is trying to come in but is crooked. This makes the chances of the permanent tooth straightening itself out greater. Obviously, this is more important for show dogs than for family pets, as the problem is cosmetic. The prognosis is *good*.

Tetracycline Staining. If any antibiotic of the tetracycline family is given to a pregnant bitch or to a puppy that is developing its permanent teeth, a yellow staining of the enamel is to be expected. (*For this reason, we do not recommend tetracycline antibiotics either in puppies under six months of age or in pregnant bitches.*)

Eye Defects

Two common eye disorders can show up by about six months of age. The first is a problem with the third eyelid and really doesn't even involve the eyeball itself. The second defect is of the retina. Each one is described here.

Cherry Eye (Prolapsing Nictitans Gland). This condition is seen most often in Cocker Spaniels. All dogs normally have three eyelids: the upper, the lower, and the third eyelid. The third eyelid is also called the *nictitans.* This eyelid sits in the inner corner of the eye and only comes up to protect the eye as needed. The nictitans has a small, fleshy gland (called the *gland of the nictitans*) on its backside. In some dogs, it flips out or protrudes and becomes visible. The owner sees this fleshy red swelling in the corner of the eye and immediately thinks the eye was damaged. This prompts a call to the vet. On examination, the veterinarian identifies the swelling as the nictitans gland. Two treatment options are available. Either the eye is treated with topical antibiotics (to guard against infection) and cortisone (to reduce swelling), or a surgical correction is performed. We occasionally see the topical medication work, but not consistently, and the gland can repeatedly prolapse. Surgery is a more permanent solution. Years ago, we used to remove this gland surgically. We now know that this gland is important for keeping the eye moist, and without it the eye can become dry.

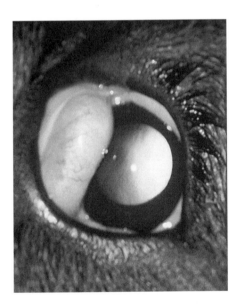

Cherry Eye is the result of a swelling and protrusion of the third eyelid (nictitans). *Dr. M. Neaderland*

The new procedure involves tacking the gland down so that it cannot continue to prolapse. I have seen this surgery performed, and the results are good and cosmetic. There is no dry-eye seen as a complication. Since this is mainly a cosmetic problem, the prognosis is *good*, with or without surgery.

Progressive Retinal Degeneration or Atrophy (PRD or PRA). This is a disorder where the retina of the eye starts to degenerate or atrophy by the time the puppy is six to twelve months of age. The reasons are genetic, and the gene has been identified as recessive in most breeds. There are several different types: PRD Type I is seen in the

Setter, Poodle, Border Collie, and Norwegian Elkhound. This degeneration is progressive, starting with poor night vision and progressing to day blindness. It can take years for complete blindness to ensue.

The PRD Type II is commonly found in working breed dogs. This form is mild compared to Type I and doesn't generally progress to complete blindness. Affected dogs retain peripheral vision, while their central vision is lost. This means objects directly in front of them will be blurred. This form may also take years to progress to a clinical state, but then stabilizes. The owner first notices a loss of vision and dilated pupils, even in bright daylight.

Diagnosis is made by a veterinarian or veterinary ophthalmologist. A *fundic* exam (examination of the fundus and retina) is performed using lenses and bright light. There are obvious changes to the retina, including atrophied optic disc, shrunken retinal blood vessels and pigmentation changes of the retina. The pupillary reflexes are usually diminished. There is no treatment, and the prevention is not to breed dogs that carry this gene. Most breeders of these dogs have the eyes of their breeding stock certified free of this defect by a veterinary ophthalmologist. This is called CERF (Canine Eye Registration Foundation). A few breeds can get either Type I or II, such as the Labrador Retriever, Border Collie, and Shetland Sheepdog. The prognosis is *fair* in Type II, but *guarded* to *poor* in Type I.

Hormonal Defects

These hormonal defects are ones that show up by six months of age. Therefore, they are associated with growth abnormalities. Since puppies generally have a growth spurt between two to six months, this is when these problems are first detected.

> *Hypothyroidism*. This literally translates to "below normal thyroid." These puppies have reduced circulating thyroid hormone. The thyroid gland, which rests in the *thoracic inlet* (where the windpipe goes into the chest), produces thyroid hormone. In these puppies, there just isn't enough. Several mechanisms can be involved, from having an underdeveloped thyroid gland to an iodine deficiency. The symptoms of congenital hypothyroidism are underdevelopment, weakness, low energy, and dwarfism. The puppy's teeth may be missing, the coat is thin and dry, and the puppy is a "poor-doer." The diagnosis is made with the clinical appearance and a thyroid blood test. The blood test measures the level of free thyroid hormone (T_4). These cases can be treated with daily thyroid hormone supplements, either natural thyroid from health

food stores or synthetic hormone in tablet form. Either way, the T_4 should be rechecked on a monthly basis until the dose is tailored to the patient. Most puppies start to thrive and flourish with the supplement. The prognosis is *fair* to *good* because the treatment works so well. By the way, the reverse condition, *hyperthyroidism*, does not occur in dogs.

Pituitary Dwarfism. The pituitary gland is a small gland that sits at the base of the brain. This kidney-bean-sized gland secretes a number of hormones that regulate several different bodily functions. One of them is body growth. In the German Shepherd Dog, Weimaraner and other German breeds, there is an inherited defect of the pituitary. It is either smaller than normal or cystic. It secretes reduced levels of growth hormone, one of the main hormones that regulate body growth. The consequence is a puppy that never grows up—a miniature version of the breed, a dwarf. The puppy may have other associated hormonal dysfunction as well. There can be mental dullness, a poor coat, an impaired immune system, immature bones, and skin defects. Diagnosis is easily made by observing the appearance of the puppy and by testing for levels of *growth hormone*. There is no cure for this condition. Treatment has been attempted with injections of growth hormone for several weeks. Growth hormone therapy is still in experimental form and very costly. Some of these puppies do respond, but due to the other concurrent hormonal problems, the prognosis is *poor*.

Muscle Defects

Muscle defects are generally seen in young puppies by their third month. Owners notice that affected puppies are tired or continually weak. They may try to run, but fall. They sometimes have trouble holding their head up. The following three conditions are quite different in their mechanisms, but may look very similar clinically. They are usually restricted to one or two breeds.

Muscular Dystrophy. This form of canine muscular dystrophy is similar to the *Duchenne* form seen in children. This defect in the X chromosome causes progressive muscle destruction throughout the body. The muscle fibers are destroyed and replaced with fat. It is seen in Golden Retriever and Irish Setter males. Symptoms of muscle weakness, abnormal gait, collapse, overextended joints, and a dropped head start at twelve weeks and progress to six months. The dogs can walk and run for only short distances before becoming weak. The heart and respiratory muscles are affected, which ultimately leads to the demise of the dog. There are high levels of a component of muscle breakdown called *creatine phosphokinase*. Diagnosis is made by the clinical presentation; a muscle biopsy, which demonstrates the muscle destruction; and elevated creatine phosphokinase levels. There is no treatment except a lot of TLC and patience. The longest any dog reported to have this affliction has lived has been six years. The prognosis is *poor*.

Myasthenia Gravis. This is a disorder of the nerve endings of the muscles. There is a lack of neurotransmitter receptors at the junction of the nerve and muscle, which leads to weakened muscle contractions. The predominant breeds affected are Springer Spaniels, and Fox and Jack Russell Terriers. Symptoms start as early as eight weeks of age, but progress until the condition is very obvious by twelve weeks. These puppies get so weak they collapse on the slightest exertion. They may have trouble swallowing and barking. A megasophagus (*see* p. 10) is commonly seen in these puppies. Diagnosis is made by observing the puppy before and after an injection of the drug Tensilon. The puppy responds almost immediately. This drug is not used as a daily treatment. Treatment with daily doses of an anticholinesterase drug is the only option other than euthanasia. The response is variable, so the prognosis is *guarded* to *poor*.

Myopathy of Labrador Retrievers. The author is personally interested in this defect. I own a black Labrador afflicted with this inherited condition. His name is Myles. Before I get into his story, let me give you some background information. Myopathy is a hereditary defect of the muscle fibers (type II) in black and yellow Labradors. Puppies start showing symptoms at three months. Most of the symptoms are of muscle weakness and atrophy. Symptoms stabilize by six months, and the dogs can make great household pets. I can use Myles as an example.

Myles was shipped to Cornell University from a breeder in 1985. He was three months old and was just starting to show signs of myopathy. I was a fourth-year student at the veterinary college, assigned to his case. His symptoms were muscle weakness and atrophy: He couldn't hold up his head, he bunny-hopped when he tried to trot, and he would collapse after walking fifty feet. He was the sweetest, kindest, most devoted puppy I had ever known. All he ever wanted was to be loved. It took Cornell nearly four months to diagnose him as a myopathy case. Muscle biopsy showed a deficiency of the type II muscle fiber, essential to prolonged muscle contractions. They put probes in his muscles to test his nerve conduction, which was normal. They tried drug therapy, which made him worse. During all this time, my wife and I would sneak him off campus to go for walks in the park. It amazed me how much he improved when outside the clinic environment. It's amazing what a little TLC will do. We named him, we took him home on weekends, we broke all the clinic rules. He was becoming ours.

Cold weather made his symptoms worse. So did excitement, as is typical. He was now six months old, and his signs were stabilizing. He could walk much farther, with short rests along the way. Since the college was finished with him—that is, they got their diagnosis—they were ready to destroy him. My wife and I couldn't allow this to happen, so we officially adopted him from the college. He is now eleven years old and doing wonderfully. He still loves his walks in the park, but now he can go a mile before he has to rest. If you can tolerate having a handicapped dog who is wonderful in every other way, then the prognosis is *great!*

Myotonia. This muscle defect is seen in the Chow Chow. It's caused by a defect in the calcium transport in the muscle, which is essential for normal contractions. This causes the muscles to stay stiff and rigid, unable to relax. Symptoms start at three to four months of age, then stabilize. The puppies jerk and appear to have muscle spasms on exertion. Diagnosis is made with a physical exam and reflex testing of specific muscle groups. This congenital defect can be confused with *tetanus*, which is a disease characterized by tetanic muscle spasms of the entire body (described in Chapter 6, "Puppy Pediatrics"). Treatment is limited to antispasmodic and muscle relaxant medications, which only help temporarily. These puppies usually do well as long as they aren't asked to do anything too athletic. Prognosis is *guarded* to *fair*.

Neurologic Defects

By the time this group of afflicted puppies is six months old, they start showing neurological symptoms. These defects are of the brain itself, the spinal cord, or the nerves that control specific functions. Symptoms of neurologic problems can manifest as weakness and paralysis; loss of balance and orientation; loss of vision, hearing, smell and touch; lack of control of limbs; muscle atrophy; tremors; and seizures. Luckily, these don't all usually occur in the same condition. Following are alphabetized descriptions of the most common neurologic conditions of six-month-old puppies.

Epilepsy. Epilepsy is defined as a condition in which regular malfunctions of the brain lead to sudden bursts of involuntary electrical activity. These bursts are called seizures or convulsions. Most cases of epilepsy in puppies are *idiopathic*, which means that the cause is unknown. The breeds most afflicted are the German Shepherd, Beagle, Poodle, Saint Bernard, Cocker Spaniel and Keeshond. Seizures come in two varieties. The first is called *petit mal*, which means "little seizure." These dogs may have only one part of their body involved, and the seizures only last moments. They are mild compared to the other type of seizure, called *grand mal*. In these cases, the entire body is involved, and the seizure can last up to ten minutes. These puppies shake, fall over, kick and paddle, lose bladder and bowel control, thrash and stiffen up. A string of grand mal seizures is called *status epilepticus*, and puppies seldom survive them.

Certain conditions and diseases can cause epilepsy in young dogs. Therefore, it is essential to rule out other causes before assuming epilepsy. The canine distemper virus is one of the most common causes of seizures in puppies. Other congenital defects can lead to seizures, such as hypoglycemia, hydrocephalus, liver disorders, portosystemic shunts, and heart disease. Toxins and heavy metal poisoning are also causes. Certain head traumas will lead to seizures, as can Lyme disease (see Chapter 2 for more details on Lyme disease).

Owners of epileptic dogs are asked to keep a log of when the seizures occur and how long they last. Your veterinarian should perform a complete physical and neurological exam. Usually blood tests are done to evaluate the internal status of the patient. If the puppy checks out normal, the diagnosis of *idiopathic epilepsy* is made. Treatment is not needed if the seizures are more than a month apart or if they last less than a minute. But if they are more frequent, most vets use an anti-epileptic drug. The most popular drugs used today are Phenobarbital and Dilantin. These help reduce the frequency and duration of the seizures but do not completely stop them. Idiopathic epilepsy has no cure. If the seizures can be managed with medication, the prognosis is *fair*.

Laryngeal Paralysis. This condition involves a slow paralysis or weakening of the larynx, or voice box. We commonly see this problem in older dogs. In puppies, we see a congenital version in the Bouvier des Flandres and the Siberian Husky. Males are the majority of the cases. Symptoms start at three to six months of age. The first symptom the owner notices is a change in the puppy's voice. It then progresses to a gasping or roaring sound during exercise-induced breathing. Breeders call this "air hunger"; medically, we call it *stridor*. What's happening is that the laryngeal nerve, which opens the larynx and voice box, is malfunctioning, consequently causing an upper airway obstruction. The cartilage flaps just don't open on one side. This phenomenon can be seen by sedating the puppy and examining the larynx with a laryngoscope.

The treatment that has worked for us is a surgical procedure that permanently ties back the collapsed cartilage, leaving it open. It is called *arytenoid lateralization*. The dog is also put on antibiotics and cortisone to reduce post-operative infection and inflammation, respectively. Common post-operative complications are coughing and scarring near the vocal cords, which can permanently make the bark hoarse. With surgery, the prognosis is good.

Lysomal Storage Disease or Gangliosidosis (GM$_{1 and 2}$). This is an inherited (autosomal recessive) neurological disease of puppies that are several months old. There is a defect of specific enzymes that are stored in sacs called *lysosomes* in nerve cells. Without these enzymes, the nerve cells cannot function properly. Clinical signs start as weakness, tremors, and can progress to seizures and paralysis. There have been several reported breeds, including setters, spaniels, pointers, small terriers, Portuguese Water Dogs, and German Shepherd Dogs. There is no treatment, and most of these puppies are euthanized by one year of age. Experimental bone marrow transplants have been tried as a way to replace the missing enzymes. There is a blood test that can detect if an animal is a carrier of the recessive gene. Definitive diagnosis usually is made by biopsy of nerve tissue. Carriers of this gene should not be used for breeding.

Skeletal Defects

Skeletal defects of young puppies were described in the last section. The following defects don't show up until close to six months of age. This is the time most normal puppies are developing and strengthening their muscles, bones and tendons. The first thing the owners notice in most of these disorders is a lack of willingness to play due to pain. Then, as the condition worsens, lameness sets in. These puppies are in obvious pain and cannot perform daily tasks without hurting. Some of the defects are worse than others. We will try to give you an idea of how serious they are and what treatments are available.

Angular Deformities. This condition is seen in breeds with long legs. Long bones of the forelimbs and hind limbs grow by elongating at both

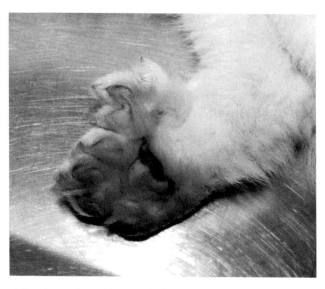

An angular deformity, such as this one of a hind leg, is a result of abnormal growth.

ends. This happens at the growth plate zones, areas at both ends of the bone that produce new bone. If one of these growth plates of a bone stops producing new bone (we call this "premature closure" of a growth plate) while the other end is still elongating, a disproportional bone will result.

If there are two bones connected at both ends (as in the radius-ulna of the forelimb, or the tibia-fibula of the hind limb), and one growth plate closes, the limb will bend or be bowed. Closure of each different growth plate will cause a different variation of angular deformities. For example, if the growth plate above the wrist of the ulna bone prematurely closes while the radius continues to grow, the forelimb will bow forward and the wrist turn outward.

If the angulation is mild, no treatment is needed. For cases involving a limp, casts or splints may be sufficient to correct the deviation. These should be used before the bones completely harden before six months of age. If the angulation is severe enough to cause a deformity of the limb, surgical treatment should be attempted by six months. The orthopedic surgeon removes a wedge of bone (called an *osteotomy*) from the curved side of the bone, then rigidly fixes the bone ends with internal hardware (like a bone plate and screws). This procedure requires great expertise and should be attempted only by a qualified surgeon. When performed correctly, a functional limb will result, although the limb may be slightly shorter than its counterpart. The prognosis is *fair* to *good* depending on the extent of the curvature and success of the surgery.

Elbow Luxation. This is a developmental defect of the elbow joint that results in a dislocated elbow (*luxated* in medical terms). This means that the three bones of the joint—the radius, the ulna, and the humerus—are not aligned. The result is an outward displacement of the elbow. It is suspected that the ligaments which hold the joint together are either underdeveloped or missing. Toy breeds are most affected. By the time the puppy is four to six months old, it is obvious to the owner that there is a problem with the limb. People say things like, "The leg just goes out on him when he runs." Diagnosis is made by clinically observing the animal as it walks and by visualizing the luxated elbow on an X ray. Treatment is surgical. The orthopedic surgeon stabilizes the joint by reconstructing the deficient ligaments or by pinning the joint. The limb is placed in a cast or splint for several weeks post-surgically. Arthritis is the most common surgical complication. The elbow is also more rigid than normal. Therefore, the prognosis is *guarded* to *fair*, depending on how much physical activity the dog will be required to do.

Fragmented Medial Coronoid Process and Elbow Dysplasia. This is a developmental flaw of the elbow joint of giant breed dogs. During development of the elbow joint, a fragment of the ulnar bone never fuses, leaving a chip-like piece of bone floating around in the elbow. Symptoms start when the puppy is as young as six months old and are painful on flexion and extension of the elbow, especially with outward rotation of the paw. There is a general instability of the joint. In other words, these dogs are lame on that limb.

The elbow may become warm and swollen. Exercise worsens the pain. The condition is diagnosed with X rays of the elbow joint in question. The detached piece of bone (coronoid process) is visualized. If left untreated, degenerative changes will occur in the elbow, ultimately leading to permanent arthritis. Splints or casts are inadequate in treating this condition. The fragmented coronoid process needs to be surgically removed. The most common side effect of surgery is arthritis. The owner needs to be aware of this and should limit exercise. The arthritis can be managed with anti-inflammatory medication such as buffered aspirin or Phenylbutazone. Due to the potential of arthritic changes down the road, the prognosis is guarded to fair with surgery.

Hip Dysplasia (HD). Hip dysplasia is the most common orthopedic deformity seen in large and giant sporting and working breeds. *Dysplasia* means "an abnormal development." This defect has an inherited origin. Many factors seem to be involved in the development of dysplasia. They include the puppy's growth rate, its muscle weight compared to bone conformation, nutritional deficiencies or over-uses, stress, excessive exercise too early in the developmental process, and other environmental factors.

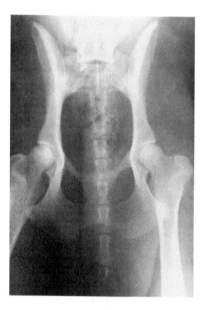

An X ray of normal hips.

The abnormal development of the hip involves all parts of this ball-in-socket joint: the acetabulum (this is the socket part), the head of the femur (this is the ball part), and the fibrous joint capsule that encompasses the joint. The deformity can be in either one or both hips. There are two components to this defect. First, there is a laxity or looseness of the joint so that the head of the femur doesn't sit inside the acetabulum properly. In dysplastic dogs, less than 50 percent of the

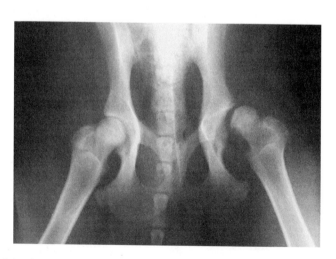

An X ray of dysplastic hips. Note how the bone on the right is out of the socket.

femoral head sits in the acetabulum. Second, as the disease progresses, a deformity of both the acetabulum and head of femur occurs. The result is instability of the hip joint, which translates into pain. These dogs have pain on manipulation, especially extension of the hip. They also experience pain when climbing up stairs, jumping, or doing anything that puts additional weight on the hindquarters.

Other symptoms include muscle atrophy of the thigh muscles, an audible "click" when the hip is adducted (the leg is raised parallel with the spine as the dog stands), a bunny-hopping gait, a stiffening of the hind legs, and more sitting than is normal.

A veterinarian diagnoses this condition by manipulating the hips, by performing certain maneuvers that demonstrate the laxity of the joint and elicit pain, and, ultimately, by taking X rays of the pelvis and hips to visualize the luxation and deformity of the joints. Most vets are qualified to diagnose hip dysplasia from the X rays, but breeders usually request confirmation by a panel of veterinary radiologists of the **Orthopedic Foundation for Animals**. X rays are sent to the foundation for an official report and rating. We call this getting an "OFA rating."

The OFA will not rate a dog under two years of age. Although symptoms may start by six months, they can progress until the dog is two years old. Studies have shown that up to 80 percent of large breed dogs show radiographic evidence of hip dysplasia by their first birthday. By the time they are two years old, 95 percent of the dogs show radiographic changes. The report is sent to both owner and referring veterinarian. The hips are rated as excellent, good, fair, borderline, or dysplastic (mild to severe). Breeders are strongly urged not to breed dogs with a dysplastic report. The radiologists look for things like roundness of femoral head, percentage of femoral head seated in acetabulum, angle of femoral neck, arthritic or degenerative changes of either femoral head or acetabulum, and a shallow acetabulum.

A new diagnostic tool for early diagnosis of hip dysplasia in dogs is called **PennHIP**. It was developed by veterinarians at the University of Pennsylvania, who found that the conventional way of x-raying hips according to the OFA technique (described above) often missed early detection of HD. According to their research, the PennHIP technique is two and a half times more sensitive at finding early joint laxity (looseness), one of the main early symptoms of hip dysplasia.

The PennHIP technique requires the dog to be put under general anesthesia, during which times three X rays are taken: a standard hip view (as done for OFA); one where the hips are stressed using a distraction device; and a third where the hips are compressed. The X ray films are viewed by a radiologist for laxity and evidence of HD. This technique can only be performed by a specially trained veterinarian. Dogs should be a minimum of four months old, and owners are advised to have them retested after one year if the procedure was done at younger than six months. Consult with your vet or breeder to see if this technique is appropriate for your puppy.

Treatments available range from mild medical attention to radical surgical correction. Mild cases can be treated with weight reduction, limited exercise, and anti-inflammatory medications such as aspirin and Phenylbutazone. Crippling cases are treated with any one of six surgical procedures, whose techniques are listed here, along with a brief description:

Pectineal Myectomy. This procedure cuts the pectineal muscle, which is implicated in causing tension in the hip joint. This surgery was more common years ago and is losing popularity. The beneficial effects are short-lived, and there is no improvement of the arthritis.

Pelvic Osteotomy. This is a complicated surgery in which the pelvis is cut and rotated to allow better seating of the femoral head into the acetabulum. This procedure should not be done if there are any degenerative changes in the joint; it only corrects a malalignment problem. It is extensive surgery; for all purposes, think of it as a pelvis reconstruction.

Femoral Osteotomy. This procedure changes the angle of the femoral head and neck so that it approaches the normal angulation. This means that the femoral head will seat better in the acetabulum. That's good. What the surgeon is doing is making the femoral neck perpendicular to the long axis of the femur shaft. This works better if there are minimal arthritic changes. The trickiest part of this surgery is determining the proper angle. There are few complications.

Total Hip Replacement. This procedure replaces the defective femoral head and acetabulum with a man-made prosthesis. The acetabulum is made from polyethylene plastic, and the femoral head is stainless steel. The dog should be allowed to reach full size prior to this surgery so that the correct size of prosthesis is chosen. This procedure is indicated when there is much degeneration of the hip. This surgery is only performed by qualified veterinary orthopedic surgeons at referral centers. The most common complications are loosening of the prosthesis, or rejection.

Femoral Head and Neck Excision. This is the most commonly performed surgery for hip dysplasia. We also perform it for hip dislocations that will not go back into joint. The philosophy with this surgery is that if the hip joint is defective, why not just remove it? This implies that a dog doesn't need a hip joint to walk on that leg. This is true to some extent. If the surgeon removes the defective head and neck of the femur, a false joint of fibrous scar tissue will form. The false joint is smoother than the rough defective one. This means that the pain from the deformed head rubbing on a deformed acetabulum is gone.

After about two months, the false joint forms, and the dog starts using the leg without pain. This procedure is indicated when there is much degeneration of the hip. We have used this technique with great success in dogs under fifty pounds. The most common complication to this surgery is a shortened leg. Postoperative physical therapy is needed to facilitate the formation of the false joint. An inexperienced surgeon may accidentally cut the *sciatic* nerve, which runs along the pelvis near where the femoral neck is removed with a chisel (osteotome). This would leave the leg permanently paralyzed.

BOP Shelf. This is a procedure used in young dogs with hip joint laxity. These hips are loose and unstable, but have no degenerative changes. The surgery involves using a composite bone material as a graft and building up the acetabular (socket) rim. This prevents the head of the femur from popping out of socket. The composite can actually stimulate natural bone growth as well. This stabilizes the joint, allowing the puppy to walk with more comfort and strength.

In mild cases, with treatment, the prognosis is *fair* to *good* for a functional pet. In severe cases, even with surgery, the prognosis is *guarded* to *poor* for returning to normal function. These dogs can still make good pets, but they need continuing special care.

Hypertrophic Osteodystrophy (HOD). This condition affects only large and giant breed dogs, especially Great Danes, Labrador Retrievers and Irish Setters. The long bones of the limbs are affected. The actual mechanism involved is as follows: When the puppy is about three to six months of age, the long bones of the limbs are growing at a maximum rate. The ends of the bones are where the new bone is made (called the growth plate or *metaphysis*), and it is from these areas that the pain emanates. The heavy weight of these large puppies causes stress to the plates, resulting in pain. The bones actually become swollen, thickened and warm. The dog reacts with pain if the bone is squeezed or pressed and may be so lame it cannot walk. The metaphysis responds by putting down more bone. This bone hardening is called *sclerosis*.

Diagnosis is made by taking a careful history of a three- to six-month-old puppy that is suffering from lameness and tender long bones. Radiographically, we can visualize the swollen (hypertrophic) growth plates with thick plate lines. A fever is often present. The treatment is twofold. First, the puppy's growth rate needs to be reduced by changing its diet. The puppy is taken off a puppy diet and placed on an adult maintenance food. All additional food supplements are stopped (this may include daily vitamins or calcium powders). Second, we make attempts to reduce the inflammation of the bone, so we prescribe anti-inflammatory drugs. These reduce swelling and pain of the bone, allowing the dog to walk. Despite these measures, the puppy has to outgrow this phase. This disappears when the bones stop growing. Most puppies spontaneously resolve by one year. The prognosis is *guarded* because these puppies are so lame, some owners request euthanasia. We find this rare, as most people are willing to wait it out.

Legg-Calvé-Perthes Disease (LCPD). This is considered the "hip dysplasia" of small breeds, though that description is not entirely accurate. LCPD is an inherited condition of breeds weighing less than fifty pounds. Yorkshire Terriers seem most prone. The process is a deterioration of the hip joint, more specifically, the femoral head and neck. The blood supply is shut off to this area. The bone cannot live without a proper blood supply, so it actually dies. This is called *avascular necrosis*, or death due to reduced blood flow. The first symptoms are the same as for hip dysplasia and start at six months. Males are more prone to this condition. These dogs have pain on manipulation, especially extension of the hip. They also experience pain when climbing up stairs, jumping, or doing anything that puts additional weight on the hindquarters. Other symptoms include muscle atrophy of the thigh muscles, an audible click when the hip is adducted (the leg is raised parallel with the spine as the dog stands), a bunny-hopping gait, a stiffening of the hind legs, and more sitting than is normal. Radiographs show the deformed, weakened femoral neck. The femoral head may also be popping out of the hip socket. All this leads to the pain these dogs are experiencing. Mild cases can be treated with analgesic and anti-inflammatory medications. More severe cases require surgery. The most successful procedure is the *femoral head and neck excision* described in detail in the "Hip Dysplasia" section. The only difference is that surgery for this disease has a higher success rate than that for hip dysplasia, most likely due to the small size of the patient.

Osteochondritis Dissecans (OCD). This is an inhereted defect of cartilage development, not bone, that affects largebreed dogs, especially the Labrador Retriever, Golden Retriever and Rottweiler. The defective cartilage actually flakes off the bone, causing pain and inflammation within the joint. The cartilage is the shock-absorbing covering to the ends of bones. It is smooth, glistening, and fibrous, and provides an excellent non-friction surface for joints. In other words, it is crucial to a properly functioning joint.

What happens in OCD is that areas of cartilage in certain joints lift off the underlying bone. These cartilage flaps cause trauma to the joint, resulting in pain and swelling of those areas, especially the shoulder, knee (stifle), hock and elbow. The diagnosis is made with X rays of the joint in question. The area of missing cartilage is seen as a translucent area on the articular surface. In most cases, the treatment is surgical removal of the cartilage flap. The remaining hole defect is *scarified* (scratched) so that scar tissue will fill in. Scar tissue isn't as good as cartilage, but it's better than nothing. At least it keeps bone from rubbing on bone, which produces pain. The prognosis is *fair*, as these dogs usually do well after surgery; however, arthritis is a common complication to joint surgery. The dog is usually on analgesics intermittently for the rest of its life and is obviously less useful for sporting purposes.

Ununited Anconeal Process (UAP). This is a lack of fusion of the anconeal process of the ulna bone to the bone shaft. During development of the bone, this process is actually detached from the main bone. It is supposed to fuse at five months of age. In the German Shepherd Dog, Labrador Retriever, Basset Hound, Saint Bernard and other large or giant breeds, this fusion never happens. What remains is a small wedged piece of bone that is free-floating in the elbow joint. At first it doesn't cause any problems, but as the puppy grows and puts more weight on the joint, stress occurs. A stressed joint is an unhappy joint. Swelling and pain ensue. The elbow becomes unstable.

These puppies are lame in the front leg. When the elbow is palpated, it appears locked. Diagnosis is confirmed with an X ray of the elbow joint, which shows the anconeal process detached from the rest of the ulna bone. Both elbows should be X-rayed because this condition can occur on both sides. The most popular treatment is to remove the detached anconeal process surgically. This allows the elbow to return to near-normal function. (A warning: Post-operative arthritis months later is an unfortunate complication of any joint surgery.) Another technique has been used in which the detached process is fixed to the main ulna with a surgical screw. These results aren't as favorable, as the process has to line up perfectly or the elbow will not bend normally. Also, screws can loosen or break when the animal puts its full weight on the joint. Therefore, we recommend the removal of the anconeal process. The prognosis is *fair* to *good*. Unfortunately, this defect is often seen in conjunction with other skeletal defects such as fragmented coronoid process/elbow dysplasia and osteochondritis dissecans (OCD).

Wobblers (Caudal Cervical Vertebral Malarticulation). This is an inherited defect of the neck vertebrae in the Doberman Pinscher and Great Dane. The sixth and seventh vertebrae have an upward displacement, which compresses the spinal cord. Any pressure on the spinal cord leads to weakness (or ataxia) of the hind, and sometimes front, legs. The dogs appear normal until about six months of age. At that time, progressive symptoms of neck pain on flexing, and weakness of the hind legs and then the front legs, become evident. There is also loss of reflexes; deep pain perception; an uncoordinated, widely swinging gait; and leg crossing when the dog walks. As the compression of the spinal cord worsens, so do the symptoms, until the dog becomes paralyzed.

Diagnosis is made with special contrast X rays of the spinal cord. This is called *contrast myelography*. In this test, the radiologist injects contrast material into the space around the spinal cord. This enables the radiologist to see just where the cord is being compressed. Views of the neck bent upward (extended) and downward (flexed) are always taken. The only permanent treatment is to eliminate the cord compression surgically and stabilize the neck. The surgery is very tricky and should be attempted only by an orthopedic veterinary surgeon. The prognosis is *guarded*, even with surgery.

Skin Defects

Two genetic defects were covered in the newborn section: hypotrichosis (genetic lack of fur) and rubber puppy syndrome (when a defect occurs in the collagen structure of the skin, making it thin, easily torn and rubbery). In fact, these defects can occur later in life, even up to six months of age. The two following defects usually do not show up until the afflicted puppy is six months of age.

Acanthosis Nigricans. This is a genetic defect of the skin of the Dachshund, which becomes evident at six months of age. I've seen some cases as late as two years, but that's unusual. The condition starts as hair loss, itching and greasy skin under the armpits and on the chest. This can progress to symmetrical hair loss under the arms, in the groin area and on the inner thighs. The skin can become quite "leathery," darkened with pigment and wrinkled. Many of these dogs are concurrently hypothyroid, which clouds the diagnosis. A thyroid blood test should always be done if this condition is suspected. A definitive diagnosis is made with a skin biopsy. Treatment consists of treating the underlying hypothyroidism (see the section on hormonal defects) and using topical medications. Vitamin E seems to help keep the skin more supple and less itchy. A new therapy involving a skin-derived hormone called *melatonin* has shown some promise when given subcutaneously. Luckily, these dogs don't go completely bald. The prognosis is generally *fair* to *good*.

Acral Mutilation. This is a sad and bizarre disorder of Pointers. For reasons that are as much neurologic as dermatologic, these dogs have increased sensation in their extremities (toes most often). This constant irritation, or increased sensitivity, drives these puppies of four to six months of age to chew at their toes. I'm not talking about mild licking and chewing; I mean complete mutilation. I've seen these dogs literally chew their toes off. They don't seem to feel their feet at all. Unfortunately, very little can be done. These dogs are absolutely determined. No amount of bandaging or sedatives seems to dissuade them. The only humane treatment is to euthanize the poor creatures before gangrene sets in. The prognosis is *grave*.

Urinary Defects

This section covers kidney and urinary bladder defects, which are sometimes difficult to distinguish. They can look the same at first. The kidney problems are usually more serious than the bladder ones. The main functions of the kidney are to reabsorb water from the blood, filter out waste products of metabolism to produce urine and regulate the concentration of body fluid salts. Since only 25 percent of the kidneys (that's only half of one kidney) is needed to sustain life, you can see that those defects which affect both kidneys are more serious than those that only affect one. The urinary bladder and the tubes that bring the urine from the kidney (called the *ureters*) are a collection and storage tank for urine. We are all aware of how important a functioning urinary bladder is!

> *Agenesis of the Kidney.* Agenesis means absence; in this case, absence of a kidney. The puppy is born with only one instead of the normal two. As mentioned in the introduction to this section, only half of one kidney is needed for life, so these puppies are not in any immediate danger. In fact, there are few symptoms at all. Recently, we saw a case of this in a German Shepherd Dog–mix puppy. The only symptom was excessive urination. Routine blood screens showed normal renal (another word for kidney) function. It wasn't until we performed an ultrasound that we discovered the dog had only one kidney. An important consideration regarding this condition is that, later in life, any problem affecting the one kidney can be life-threatening because no backup kidney exists. Therefore, urinary infections must be treated quickly and aggressively in order to prevent complications. No other treatment is needed. The prognosis is generally *good.*

> *Dysplasia of Kidney.* This means an abnormally developed kidney. It is seen in many breeds, including the Lhasa Apso, Shih Tzu, Alaskan Malamute, Doberman Pinscher, Norwegian Elkhound, Poodle and Soft Coated Wheaten Terrier. The kidney is small, deformed and hardened, and it doesn't function normally. Since this kidney is basically useless, the puppy functions as if it had only one kidney. Therefore, the symptoms, diagnosis, treatment and prognosis are similar to those just discussed in "Agenesis of the Kidney."

> *Ectopic Ureter.* This is a condition of young female dogs, especially the Siberian Husky and Golden Retriever. The ureter is the tube that connects the kidney to the urinary bladder. Newly made urine flows from the kidney through the ureter into the bladder, where it collects until the animal urinates. The word "ectopic" means "located at an abnormal position." Therefore, an ectopic ureter means that it goes somewhere it shouldn't. In these cases, it bypasses the urinary bladder and empties directly into the vaginal tract, or uterus. The condition usually occurs only on one side. The problem is that since urine is

constantly being made by the kidneys, urine is continually flowing down the ureters. On the normal side the urine dumps into the urinary bladder, but on the ectopic side it flows directly into the vagina and then dribbles down the legs. Affected puppies don't seem to have control over their urination. We call this *urinary incontinence.*

When the puppy is young, the owner may think this normal, since the puppy isn't housebroken yet. But by the time the puppy is four to six months of age, it becomes clear there is a problem. Diagnosis is made with a careful history of the puppy's incontinence and contrast X rays (called *excretory urography*) showing the dilated ectopic ureter, or by endoscopy of the vaginal tract. In the latter case, a small endoscope is threaded up the vaginal tract to where the ureter's opening is. The vet performing the procedure can then see it. Another tool to visualize the ectopic ureter is ultrasound. Treatment is always surgical. The ectopic ureter literally has to be "reimplanted," or put back into the bladder. Postoperatively, antibiotics are given to avoid kidney or urinary bladder infections. Unfortunately, many of these patients continue to be incontinent even after surgery. Therefore, the prognosis is *guarded.*

Hypospadias. This is a defect of the penis in young male puppies. Instead of the penis having a hole in the tip for the urine to flow out of, it has a hole on the underside. The owners notice that the dog is always wet with urine and doesn't have a good urine stream when he urinates. The dog will lick himself constantly to try to clean up the leaking urine. This defect is a nuisance and can allow bacteria to enter the urinary bladder. There may be a concurrent urinary bladder infection, which would require antibiotics and urine acidifiers. Diagnosis is made during a physical exam. The veterinarian may notice the wetness under the penis, then will actually see the hole. Treatment is surgical closure of the hole in the penile urethra so that the urine flows through the penile tip. If this is the only defect, the prognosis is *good*; however, hypospadias can occur with other defects of the penis and sheath, in which case it is *guarded.*

Nephropathy. In this inherited condition, both kidneys are deformed and nonfunctional. There are theories that the kidneys never properly develop. The two breeds we see this in are the Lhasa Apso and the Shih Tzu. These puppies start showing signs of a chronic renal failure by three to six months of age. Weight loss, anemia, vomiting, a urinal smell to the breath and high blood urea nitrogen and creatinine levels are diagnostic. X rays and ultrasounds show the small fiberoptic scarred kidneys. Rarely do we have to go to kidney biopsy for a diagnosis: The pups usually die before they are a year old. No cure exists (dialysis and kidney transplants for dogs are still only experimental). The prognosis is *poor* to *grave*.

Patent Urachus and Diverticulum. The urachus is a tube that connects the urinary bladder to the umbilical cord (navel) in the fetus. This canal normally closes within a few days of birth. In some puppies, it doesn't. These puppies can actually dribble urine from their navel. This opening is a constant source of infection for the urinary bladder in the puppy. Sometimes these canals end in a blind cyst we call a *diverticulum*. Therefore, the bladder is not smooth because of this bulging at the tip. It becomes a site for bacteria and crystals to accumulate.

Although you would think the problem would be detected early, many people don't recognize it until their second or third vet visit. A contrast cystogram X ray is needed to visualize the urachus and deformed urinary bladder. The correction of this defect is surgical ligation (tying off) of the fetal tube and, sometimes, reconstruction of the urinary bladder. This is usually done at the time of spaying or neutering. Antibiotics are given pre- and postoperatively to guard against infection. These puppies do well and, at worst, have a minor recurrent bladder infection. The prognosis is *good*.

Polycystic Kidney. Polycystic means "many cysts." A *cyst* is a fluid-filled sac or bubble. Therefore, a polycystic kidney is one that has many fluid-filled sacs. This kidney defect is the most common. Since only one kidney is cystic, there are no clinical signs. In fact, it may go undiagnosed for months to years before it is discovered incidentally. The cystic kidney is larger than the normal kidney and irregular in shape. It may be noticed during a routine physical exam or on an abdominal X ray. Sometimes we notice them during spaying. The only treatment is for severe cases where the cysts become so large that the kidney has to be surgically removed. We call this surgery *nephrectomy*. As long as the other kidney is normal, the prognosis is *good*.

Urolithiasis. This literally means "stones in the urine." We usually see it as a condition in middle-aged dogs, but it can also occur in young puppies. These stones (also called *calculis*) form either in the kidney or the urinary bladder, the latter being more common. A defect occurs in the filtration of these salts in the kidney, so an abnormally high amount of them end up in the urine. Two breeds are known for this problem: Miniature Schnauzers and Dalmatians. They are different in that they form different kinds of stones. Schnauzers tend to form *struvite* stones. Male Dalmatians form *urate* stones. There are other stone types that can form in any breed, such as *calcium oxalate*.

Symptoms are straining to urinate, blood in the urine and frequent urinations of small amounts. This condition can manifest when the puppy is as young as eight to twelve weeks of age. A urinalysis test shows the presence of the crystals and/or stones in the urine. If the stones are the size of a pea or larger, they can be seen on an X ray and should be removed surgically. Ultrasound will show stones as small as grains of sand. This sediment irritates the lining of the urinary bladder, causing a bladder infection. Urolithiasis only becomes life-threatening if there is an obstruction to the outflow of urine. Most veterinarians refer to this as the patient being "blocked." Obstructive urolithiasis occurs most commonly in the male where the stones lodge in the out-flow pipe of the penis (called the *urethra*). We occasionally see it in females. Other factors that affect stone and crystal formation are bacteria levels in the bladder, and urine pH. Urine pH is a measure of how acidic the urine is. Normally, the pH should be below 7. A pH greater than 7 encourages struvite stone formation but dissolves calcium oxalate.

Treatment can include surgical removal of notable stones; antibiotics; urine acidifiers, which lower the pH of the urine and help dissolve struvite stones; and special "prescription diets" that are low in mineral content and can help dissolve the stones or crystals. These diets are used for a short time only, and are available through veterinarians. Cases tend to be recurrent, however, so the puppy may need to be kept on a diet restricted in magnesium, phosphorus and calcium to cut down on the relapses. The prognosis is fair to good, depending how severe the case is.

Alphabetical List of Congenital and/or Inherited Defects by Age Group.
Defects Noticed at Birth

1. Cleft Palate and Harelip
2. Hermaphrodites, or Intersexing
3. Imperforate Anus
4. Skeletal Defects
   a. Hydrocephalus
   b. Open Fontanel
   c. Spina Bifida
   d. Swimmers (Flat Puppy Syndrome)

5. Skin Disorders
   a. Acquired Skin Diseases of Newborns
   b. Hypotrichosis
   c. Rubber Puppy Syndrome
6. Stillborn
7. Umbilical and Inguinal Hernias

Defects Noticed by Eight Weeks of Age

1. Anovaginal Fistulae
2. Dental Defects
   a. Absence of Teeth
   b. Enamel Defects
   c. Overshot and Undershot Jaw
   d. Supernumerary Teeth
   e. Split Twin Crown
3. Digestive Defects
   a. Dysphagia
   b. Megaesophagus
   c. Pancreatic Insufficiency
   d. Persistent Right Aortic Arch
4. Ear Defects
   a. Cauliflower Ear
   b. Deafness
5. Eye Defects
   a. Collie Eye
   b. Corneal Opacities
   c. Dermoids
   d. Distichiasis
   e. Ectropion
   f. Entropion
   g. Iris Cysts
   h. Juvenile Cataracts
   i. Night Blindness
   j. Persistent Pupillary Membrane (PPM)
   k. Retinal Dysplasia
6. Heart Defects
   a. Aortic Stenosis
   b. Pulmonic Stenosis
   c. Patent Ductus Arteriosus (PDA)
   d. Ventricular Septal Defect (VSD)
7. Hormonal Defects
   a. Hypoglycemia
   b. Juvenile Diabetes Mellitus
8. Liver Defects
   a. Copper Storage Disease of Bedlington and West Highland White Terriers
   b. Glycogen Storage Disease
   c. Portosystemic Shunts (PSS)

9. Neurological Defects

    a. Cerebellar Hypoplasia

    b. Narcolepsy

    c. Vestibular Disorders

10. Respiratory Defects

    a. Collapsing Trachea

    b. Diaphragmatic Hernia

    c. Emphysema

    d. Stenotic Nares

11. Trick Knees

12. Undescended Testicles

Defects Noticed by Six Months of Age

1. Blood Abnormalities

    a. Autoimmune Hemolytic Anemia (AIHA)

    b. Aplastic Anemia

    c. Polycythemia

    d. Thrombocytopenia

    e. Von Willebrand's Disease (VWD)

2. Dental Defects

    a. Teething

    b. Retained Deciduous Teeth

    c. Tetracycline Staining

3. Eye Defects

    a. Cherry Eye (Prolapsing Nictitans Gland)

    b. Progressive Retinal Degeneration or Atrophy (PRD or PRA)

4. Hormonal Defects

    a. Hypothyroidism

    b. Pituitary Dwarfism

5. Muscle Defects

    a. Muscular Dystrophy

    b. Myasthenia Gravis

    c. Myopathy of Labrador Retrievers

    d. Myotonia

6. Neurologic Defects

    a. Epilepsy

    b. Laryngeal Paralysis

    c. Lysosomal Storage Disease

7. Skeletal Defects

    a. Angular Deformities

    b. Elbow Luxation

    c. Fragmented Medial Coronoid Process and Elbow Dysplasia

    d. Hip Dysplasia (HD)

    e. Hypertrophic Osteodystrophy (HOD)

    f. Legg-Calvé-Perthes Disease

    g. Osteochondritis Dissecans (OCD)

    h. Ununited Anconeal Process (UAP)

    i. Wobblers (Caudal Cervical Vertebral Malarticulation)

8. Skin Defects

    a. Acanthosis Nigricans

    b. Acral Mutilation

9. Urinary Defects

    a. Agenesis of the Kidney

    b. Dysplasia of Kidney

    c. Ectopic Ureter

    d. Hypospadias

    e. Nephropathy

    f. Patent Urachus and Diverticulum

    g. Polycystic Kidney

    h. Urolithiasis

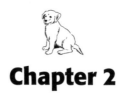

Chapter 2

All About Vaccines

This chapter is concerned with the vaccinations available for your new puppy. The definition of a vaccine is "a suspension of pieces of infectious organisms (bacteria or virus) that are administered to an animal for the prevention of that infectious disease." In other words, the vaccines must be given *prior* to exposure to the disease in order for them to work. Other names for *vaccine* are *immunization*, *shot* and *vaccination*. There are many different types of vaccines. The ones most often used in veterinary medicine are outlined next.

Types of Vaccines

Killed or inactivated vaccine. These vaccines are made of killed virus particles. The virus is killed by various means, then made into a suspension. They are generally safe, mild vaccines, but may not be as effective as the *modified live* vaccines.

Attenuated or modified live. These vaccines are made from live bacteria or viruses that have been treated so as to lose their virulence (the capability to cause disease).

Autogenous. A vaccine made from the actual organisms cultured from the animal for which the vaccine is intended. This type is used for wart vaccines.

Bacterial or Bacterin. These vaccines are made from pieces of infectious bacteria.

Nosode. This is an oral vaccine made from by-products of animals infected by that same disease. In other words, the vaccine is made from the tissues of an animal suffering from that same disease. For example, a distemper nosode would be made from substances from an animal with distemper. These vaccines are generally used by homeopathic veterinarians.

Polyvalent. These vaccines are made from several different strains of the infectious organism.

How Vaccines Work

The theory behind a vaccine is quite complex. But in simple terms, what we are doing when we give a vaccine is administering those parts of an infectious organism (bacteria or virus) that stimulate an immune response from the host (the animal getting the shot). The host's body makes antibodies, which are proteins made by the immune system that circulate in the blood, to match the small antigens (proteins on the surface of the organism) in the vaccine. What do these antibodies do? They combine with their corresponding antigens whenever they come in contact with one. When millions of antibodies are combined with the antigens found on the surface of bacteria or viruses, these organisms are rendered inactive and are incapable of causing disease. By being coated with a layer of antibody proteins, a bacterium or virus is *inactivated*. This is how a vaccine prevents disease. The key word here is *prevents*. Most vaccines only work if given before exposure to the disease. Occasionally, veterinarians use vaccines to boost the immune response in an animal suffering from a disease, as a form of treatment. This procedure is a bit controversial and is not the main intent of vaccine usage.

Not all infectious diseases have vaccines available. In fact, of the hundreds of infectious diseases of dogs, only a handful of vaccines are currently on the market. Luckily, or by design, the vaccines available are for the most common diseases of dogs. Here is a list of canine diseases for which vaccines are available.

- Canine Distemper
- Leptospirosis
- Adenovirus Type-1 or -2
- Parainfluenza
- Canine Parvovirus

These viruses are usually combined into a five-in-one vaccine, abbreviated $DA_{1-2}LP\text{-}P$ or **DHLP-P.**

- *Bordetella bronchiseptica* (Kennel Cough)
- Borreliosis (Lyme Disease)
- Canine Coronavirus
- Rabies

These vaccines are available separately or in combinations. We generally use the DHLP-P distemper vaccine and "split-out" (give individually) the other vaccines. Occasionally breeders will ask us to split-out the Distemper-Leptospirosis-Adenovirus-Parainfluenza from the Parvovirus. The thought is that a purer form of the vaccine is in the individual form. Also, with the parvovirus given individually, the vet has the choice of using a killed or modified live vaccine. This in turn produces better immunity and fewer side effects. This has not been proven scientifically, but enough veterinarians have noticed this anecdotally to warrant giving the procedure some consideration.

How Vaccines Are Given

There are three different ways to administer vaccines to animals. They can be given by subcutaneous injection, by intramuscular injection or by intranasal route. These methods are described in the following sections. Each vaccine has an approved mode of administration, as determined by the Food and Drug Administration (FDA). This organization also licenses the vaccine for a specific duration—one year, two years or three years. For example, a one-year vaccine is considered expired one year from the date of administration.

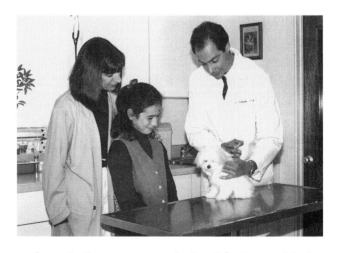

There are several ways to give a puppy a vaccination. Subcutaneous injection, as shown here, is the most common. *Donna DeBitetto*

Subcutaneous Injection

The veterinarian injects the vaccine under the skin of the animal, usually in the loose skin of the scruff area of the neck. This area naturally has fewer nerve endings than other areas, so the dog doesn't feel the vaccine as much. There is no post-vaccine soreness (although mild itching can occur), and it is an easily accessible area. This is the most common way of giving a vaccine.

Intramuscular Injection

The veterinarian injects the vaccine into a muscle. It is generally thought that intramuscular injections enter the bloodstream quicker than subcutaneous ones, and can stimulate a stronger immune response. There can often be muscle soreness for a day or two post-vaccine. Some vaccines are required to be given this way.

Intranasal Administration

These vaccines are not given by injection, but rather in the form of nose drops. Only one vaccine (*Bordetella bronchiseptica*) is currently available in this form for dogs. These vaccines start a very strong and effective immune reaction locally. Since the *Bordetella bronchiseptica* organism enters through the upper respiratory tract, the local immunity there is very effective in stopping the disease.

Why Should I Vaccinate?

Your veterinarian will be more than happy to expound on all the reasons why you should vaccinate your new puppy. Chances are, whether you obtained your puppy from a shelter, pet store or breeder, it received at least one vaccine before you brought it home. All dogs are susceptible to these diseases. If their mother had immunity to them through vaccinations, the puppy will too for several weeks. This passive transfer of immunity from the dam (mother) to the puppy occurs at two different times: first, in utero while the fetus is developing; and second, through the first nursing of the dam's first milk (we call this immunity-rich milk *colostrum*). Unfortunately, this passive immunity is short-lived compared to the immunity the puppy actively makes from a vaccine. The mother's antibodies are only intended to get the puppy off on the right paw. After about ten to sixteen weeks (the average being about twelve weeks), this immunity disappears, leaving the puppy susceptible to these diseases should it contact them. If the owner doesn't follow up with vaccinations, the puppy is at a higher risk of developing these diseases.

Vaccines By Type, Administration and Duration			
Vaccine	Type	Route of Administration	Duration in Years
Canine Distemper-Leptospirosis-Adenovirus-Parainfluenza	MLV	SC	1
Canine Parvovirus	MLV, K	SC	1
Bordetella bronchiseptica	MLV	IN	1
Borreliosis (Lyme)	K	IM	1
Canine Coronavirus	K	SC	1
Rabies	K	SC, IM	1-3

MLV= Modified Live Virus, **K=** Killed Virus, **SC=** Subcutaneous, **IN=** Intranasal, **IM=** Intramuscular

When Should I Vaccinate?

The vaccine schedule is the age and interval in which we vaccinate puppies. The age we start vaccinating is dictated by how long the dam's immunity lasts. Why? Because the maternal antibodies to a specific disease combine with the vaccine, neutralizing it. This means the vaccine didn't take and won't stimulate any immunity from the puppy's own immune system. From this, you can see that we must wait for the maternal immunity to disappear before we can expect our vaccine to work. The problem is that different maternal antibodies last different times. And each mother's immunity is different. That is, the time it takes for the dam's immunity to fall off varies greatly from puppy to puppy. We have learned through testing that most maternal antibodies last anywhere from two to twenty weeks. In 30 percent of puppies, maternal antibodies are gone after the puppy is nine to ten weeks old. Over 90 percent of the mother's immunity is gone after the puppy is sixteen weeks old. Therefore, we have developed vaccine schedules to fit the average case. The basic principles of vaccination are listed here:

- Start vaccinations as young as two to four weeks of age if the puppy was orphaned and did not have any of the mother's first milk (colostrum).

- If you start vaccinating before the puppy is eight weeks old, consider these vaccines temporary and start the puppy series at eight weeks.

- Vaccinate for those diseases that are endemic in your area (ask your vet which they are).

- If the puppy is living in close proximity to other dogs or is going to be exposed to other dogs at training classes, the groomer's, dog shows or neighborhood play groups, vaccination should start promptly when the puppy is eight weeks of age.

- The DHLP-P vaccine is given every three to four weeks until the puppy reaches sixteen weeks.

- Most states where rabies is endemic require a rabies vaccine between three to six months of age for licensing of the dog.

- Rarely, we see puppies allergic to the components of the vaccine, so monitor puppies for twenty minutes after vaccination for any signs of an allergic reaction.

- Booster the vaccine at the specified interval, usually every one to three years, to keep the level of immunity protective.

Why Booster the Vaccines?

The antibodies that the vaccines stimulate have a definite life span. Generally, modified live vaccines produce longer-lasting immunity than killed vaccines. When a vaccine gets licensed by the Food and Drug Administration, it gets licensed for a specified period. This means that the antibodies last and will be protective for that period. Most of the vaccines licensed today are for one year. This means that the veterinarian needs to revaccinate yearly. This revaccination process is called *boostering*. By doing so, the animal regenerates immunity to the disease and remains protected. Conversely, if the owner forgets to booster, the immunity lapses and the dog becomes susceptible. So, when you get a reminder card from your vet about your dog's vaccines, don't just toss it into the circular file!

Are There Any Drawbacks to Vaccines?

We mentioned earlier the two types of reactions we occasionally see in puppies, which are vaccine reactions (mild and more common) and allergy anaphylactic reactions (very serious and rare).

Another drawback is something called "vaccine failure." It means just what it says. For certain reasons, the vaccine just doesn't "take" (produce immunity), leaving the puppies susceptible to disease. There is nothing more frustrating for a veterinarian than to have a puppy come down with a disease that the puppy had already been vaccinated against. There are many reasons why a vaccine might not work:

Puppy Vaccine Schedule						
Vaccine	8 weeks	12 weeks	16 weeks	20 weeks	yearly	semi-annually
Distemper DHLP-P	X	X	X		X	
Canine Parvovirus	X	X	X	X	X	
Canine Coronavirus	X	X	X		X	
Bordetella (Kennel Cough)		X			X	X
Borreliosis (Lyme)			X	X	X	
Rabies			X		X	

- Each animal is different and has a different immune system. Therefore, the response from it will vary from dog to dog. This concept is called biological variation.

- If the dam's immunity lasts longer than the normal sixteen weeks, subsequent vaccines will not take.

- The vaccine had expired.

- The vaccine was administered improperly; i.e., an intramuscular vaccine was given subcutaneously.

- Nothing is 100 percent. Vaccines generally approach 90 to 95 percent efficacy.

- The puppy was on high doses of cortisone medication, which suppresses immune responses when vaccinated.

- The puppy was immunosuppressed by disease, stress, malnutrition or heavy parasitism when vaccinated, and could not procedure an immune response.

Vaccine Diseases

The diseases vaccines are made to protect against are some of the worst, most serious diseases of dogs. It would make sense that the most money and time spent in the research and development of a vaccine would go to those diseases that caused the most sickness and suffering to the largest population of dogs. Following is a summary of the diseases of the common vaccines on the market. New vaccines are in development all the time at animal pharmaceutical companies and veterinary colleges. Most of the vaccines available on the market today are for diseases that have plagued the canine kingdom for centuries. The most recent addition is the *Borrelia burgdorferi* or Lyme vaccine. Assume that all puppy diseases are not contagious to people, unless otherwise stated.

Canine Distemper

This is a viral disease of dogs that is highly contagious to other dogs. It is in the same family of viruses as human measles. First noticed at the turn of the century, it was believed to be a respiratory disease. This is because the virus first causes upper respiratory symptoms, then produces digestive and, ultimately, neurologic symptoms. Dogs become infected with the virus through the upper respiratory tract: eyes, nose and throat. Dogs become infected by contact with contaminated feces, saliva and sputum from infected dogs. The incubation period is about four to nine days.

The first clinical signs are fever, conjunctivitis, sneezing, coughing and labored breathing. There is often a thick pus discharge from the eyes and nose. Pneumonia is common. This can last for one to two weeks. At this point, the dog goes into a digestive tailspin. Vomiting and diarrhea start, causing weight loss and dehydration. Of the dogs who survive this stage, about 50 percent go on to develop neurological symptoms, which can include blindness, circling, falling over, tremors and seizures. Dogs with neurological symptoms are in critical condition. The virus actually invades the brain and spinal cord tissues.

Diagnosis is made by observing these classic symptoms and by taking a blood titer test, which tests the level of antibodies to the virus. Pathology tests can detect the actual viral particles in the nerve tissue. If the puppy was recently vaccinated for distemper, the titer results need to be interpreted carefully. There is no treatment for a virus other than supportive care. This means hospitalization. Antibiotics are often given to control secondary infection. Even with twenty-four-hour care and aggressive supportive therapy, the prognosis is *poor* to *grave*. The best prevention is early vaccination and minimal exposure to other strange dogs. Distemper is the **D** in DHLP-P.

Canine Adenovirus Type-1 (Infectious Hepatitis)

This is another contagious virus of dogs. It doesn't cause neurological symptoms like the distemper virus; instead, it causes an inflammation of the liver, something called *hepatitis*. The virus is spread through bodily fluids of an infected dog. The virus enters through the upper respiratory tract, and the incubation period is two to five days. The virus targets the kidneys and liver. The liver is damaged from the infection two to three weeks into the infection.

The first symptom is a nonspecific fever. It progresses to loss of appetite, vomiting, abdominal pain, and an inflamed liver. Occasionally jaundice (a yellowing of the body tissues) is seen, a classic symptom of liver damage. Some dogs also develop a cloudiness or hazing to the cornea (surface of the eye). This is called "blue eye." Diagnosis is difficult, due to the vagueness of the symptoms. A blood chemistry test shows elevations of the liver enzymes, indicating liver impairment. So does a raised bile acid blood test. Ultrasounds of the abdomen can show an enlarged liver. These findings, in combination with a high persistent fever, point to the diagnosis of adenovirus Type-1. Autopsy pathology biopsies show liver necrosis (dead tissue). Viral particles can be identified.

Treatment is supportive, since there is no cure for a virus. Medications can reduce liver inflammation. Antibiotics are often given to control secondary infection. Those dogs that survive the initial disease can have chronic liver damage or permanent eye impairment. Prevention through vaccination is recommended. We recommend using the killed vaccines because the modified live vaccines have been known to have side effects in the eye similar to the corneal damage seen in the actual disease process. The other alternative is to use a vaccine that uses the adenovirus type-2 strain, because this also protects against the type-1, but without the side effects. The prognosis is *poor* due to the serious nature of liver disease. Adenovirus type-1 is the **H** in DHLP-P.

Canine Adenovirus Type-2

This virus is another strain of the adenovirus just described. It causes a respiratory disease rather than a liver disease. Many research scientists feel that this virus can occur alone or in combination with other organisms to cause kennel cough (scientifically known as *infectious tracheobronchitis*). Respiratory viruses enter the body through the upper respiratory tract: eyes, nose and throat. Within several days, symptoms develop, which include sneezing, nasal discharge, coughing, wheezing, runny eyes and labored breathing. There is always the danger of secondary bacterial bronchial infections and pneumonia.

Treatment consists of antibiotics for secondary bacterial infections, use of cough suppressants and supportive measures. Decongestants and expectorants are helpful if there is mucus production. The virus usually runs its course in a couple of weeks, though we have seen these cases go into chronic bronchitis. Therefore, the prognosis is *guarded*. Adenovirus type-2 is a variation of the **H** in DHLP-P.

Leptospirosis

This disease is caused by the *Leptospira* organism, which is a spirochete (a corkscrew-shaped bacterium). These organisms enter the body through the mucous membranes, such as the mouth, conjunctiva and genitals. The bacteria invade the blood vessels of the liver, kidneys and urinary bladder. The incubation period is one to two weeks. The dogs have a high fever (102° to 104°F), body aches, vomiting, loss of appetite, nosebleeds, abdominal pain, uveitis (inflammation of the inside eye), liver enlargement, blood in stool and jaundice (a yellowing of the mucous membranes and skin). If the case is severe, the dog may die suddenly. More commonly, the cases are milder and chronic.

Diagnosis is made through observation of the clinical signs; serum chemistry blood tests, which show liver failure; cultures of urine, which may grow the *Leptospira* organisms; and a technique called dark field microscopy. This is where the organism is visualized in a fresh urine sample, using a dark background under the microscope. Blood titers can follow a rise in antibodies to the spirochete, implicating it as the organism.

Once the diagnosis is made, treatment is started immediately. Large doses of antibiotics are given for several weeks. Complete recovery can be expected, but those patients with liver and/or kidney damage may be chronically affected. Therefore, the prognosis is *guarded*. Prevention with a vaccine is advised if this disease is in your area. Leptospirosis is the **L** in DHLP-P.

Canine Parainfluenza

Think of this as a flu virus of dogs. It is very similar to the adenovirus type-2 described previously. It causes a respiratory infection of the upper respiratory tract and sometimes the bronchi and lungs. Many research scientists feel this virus can occur alone or in combination with other organisms to cause kennel cough (scientifically known as *infectious tracheobronchitis*). The virus gains entry into the body through the nose, throat and eyes. The incubation period is short, being about nine days. Sneezing, runny nose and eyes, and coughing are common signs, and the dog usually runs a fever. Treatment with antibiotics to guard against secondary bacterial infection, and use of decongestants and cough suppressants with an expectorant are also useful. The prognosis is *good*. The parainfluenza virus can be seen in combination with other respiratory diseases. In adults, the virus isn't that serious, but in puppies, it can cause high morbidity. Parainfluenza is the first **P** in DHLP-P.

Canine Parvovirus

This virus is one of the newest to hit the dog world. It was first discovered in 1978 in the United States. This new virus hits like a ton of bricks. All of a sudden puppies experience explosive enteritis (intestinal infection) and cardiac complications. Many die suddenly. Autopsies reveal widespread destruction and hemorrhage of the intestinal tract and cardiac muscle. Puppies less than twelve weeks of age are hit the hardest. Symptoms are sudden, explosive, watery, foul and bloody diarrhea that won't respond to any medical treatment. There are generally high fevers and acute abdominal pain. Vomiting is also persistent. This virus is highly contagious through fecal contamination. It is thought to be a major factor in the *fading puppy syndrome*, where young newborns die within their first week of life for unknown reasons.

This virus is a complicated one. More than one strain of parvovirus exists. There is the original strain first diagnosed in 1978, and a newer, variant strain that accounts for most cases seen today. Not all vaccines available have both strains, or even the newer variant. Check with your veterinarian to find the parvovirus vaccine that will protect your puppy the best. Newer vaccines out now can boast higher concentrations of the new strain. Luckily, the older vaccine is protective against both strains.

Diagnosis is made by observing the clinical signs and by giving diagnostic blood tests. A serum titer will show elevated antibody levels to the parvovirus. Experimentally, the virus can be identified in the feces by electron microscopy. There is also a fetid odor to the feces, which is very characteristic of the disease. Veterinarians try desperately to treat these cases, in which the puppies are in shock and are dehydrating quickly due to the amount of fluid loss from the diarrhea. We use intravenous fluids to replace lost body fluids, antibiotics, antispasmodics, electrolyte replacements and vitamins, but to little benefit. Over half the cases in young puppies are lost. Adults have a milder form and have a much better prognosis. Those puppies that do survive can have permanent heart damage to the myocardial muscle. The prognosis for young puppies is *poor*. The best prevention is to vaccinate all puppies for parvovirus as part of the distemper five-in-one vaccine. Ask your veterinarian which vaccine is best for your puppy. Parvovirus is the second **P** in DHLP-P.

Canine Coronavirus

This is another intestinal virus of dogs. It is not as devastating as the parvovirus just described. The average case of coronavirus starts as vomiting and intractable diarrhea, and there is usually fever. The diarrhea is not as watery as seen in parvovirus, but is light-colored and occasionally bloody. It also lacks that fetid odor. As in parvovirus, the feces are infectious to other dogs. The treatment is the same as for parvovirus: intravenous fluids, antibiotics, antispasmodics, electrolyte replacements and vitamins. There is a much higher success rate in coronavirus cases. Only the very young and debilitated puppies don't survive. For the average case, the prognosis is *fair*. Prevention is accomplished with a killed coronavirus vaccine given at eight, twelve, and sixteen weeks.

Bordetella Bronchiseptica

This bacterium is thought to be the main component of the *infectious tracheobronchitis* complex of diseases know as kennel cough. As mentioned previously, two other common agents occur simultaneously with *B. bronchiseptica* to cause kennel cough: adenovirus type-2 and canine parainfluenza virus. These three agents, when in combination, cause kennel cough. This disease is characterized by sudden bouts of a dry, hacking, persistent cough that sounds like a goose honking. The dog literally stays up at night coughing. This in turn keeps the owner up and prompts a call to the vet. The incubation period for *B. bronchiseptica* is three to four days after exposure. This bacterium is extremely contagious and becomes airborne, meaning the bacteria actually float in the air on saliva, nasal and sputum droplets, and infect dogs in the immediate area. In fact, this disease is so common in boarding kennels, it was named for it. In truth, the disease is common anywhere dogs congregate, like vets' offices, dog shows, parks, the groomer's and training classes.

Kennel cough comes in two forms: uncomplicated and complicated. Uncomplicated kennel cough refers to an average case of the disease, in which the dog coughs for one to two weeks and spontaneously gets better. We still treat these cases with antibiotics and cough suppressants. There are no complications in this form. The second, complicated form is more severe. These cases start off the same as the uncomplicated ones, but the symptoms linger beyond two weeks.

The dogs most prone to this are the very young or old and those dogs with upper respiratory problems such as collapsing trachea, pushed-in faces, allergies, asthma and congenital defects of the bronchial tubes (see Chapter 1). The complications are either chronic bronchitis or bacterial pneumonia. The bacterial organism most often cultured from these cases is *B. bronchiseptica*. The cultures are obtained by retrieving tracheal and bronchial secretions from the patient under anesthesia by infusing sterile saline water down the trachea, and then suctioning some back. This retrieves bronchial secretions with the bacteria. This procedure is called *tracheal wash*. We have treated cases of secondary pneumonia and bronchitis for several months after the onset of kennel cough, qualifying it as a chronic disease.

The *B. bronchiseptica* bacteria are tenacious and cling to the mucosal lining of the respiratory tract, making the bacteria difficult to eliminate. In a case of kennel cough, the body's immune system produces antibodies to the causative agents. This natural immunity imparted from an infection lasts only several months, which means the same puppy could get the disease again several months later if re-exposed.

The prognosis for the uncomplicated form is *good*, whereas for the complicated one it's *guarded* to *poor*. The best prevention for kennel cough is to vaccinate several days prior to going into the kennel. The most popular form of vaccine is an intranasal vaccine. The vaccine stimulates a local immune response in the upper respiratory tract, where the bacteria and viruses gain access to the body. This immune response has been shown to be very effective as a preventive. Although most of these vaccines are licensed for a year, we recommend a booster semiannually.

Rabies

Just the name of this virus strikes fear into the heart of most people. The Disney movie *Old Yeller* was a depiction of how horrible this disease is (rabies was called *hydrophobia* in the movie). This virus can infect all mammals. There is almost a 100 percent fatality rate. People are also susceptible. All puppies should be vaccinated for rabies starting at three to four months of age, and boostered routinely. Many states have laws requiring rabies vaccines of all dogs. Rabies' natural hosts are wildlife such as foxes, skunk, raccoons and, especially, bats. Each state regulates this disease by keeping data and tracking certain wildlife species. Certain countries don't have rabies, and trying to ship an animal there usually involves a lengthy quarantine. England, for example, has a six-month quarantine for an animal being shipped that originates from a rabies-endemic country.

Your pet can become infected with rabies by being bitten by a rabid animal. The virus is shed from the infected animal's saliva. It can also be spread from saliva contamination of open wounds. Therefore, if your puppy comes home with an obvious wound, and saliva or blood on its fur, put on protective gloves before handling the dog. The incubation period is variable—weeks to months. Clinical signs usually start two to three weeks after exposure, but can be as long as three months. The classic symptoms are neurologic. The virus enters the body through the wound or bite and travels along nerves until it reaches the central nervous system, spinal cord and brain. It then settles in the salivary glands.

Obvious signs are sudden behavioral changes; sudden aggression; paralysis of the jaw, which leads to the classic "foaming at the mouth"; circling; blindness; incoordination; change of voice; and seizures. Due to the gravity of this disease and its public health significance, if a dog is suspected of rabies, it is quarantined by the applicable health department. If it dies within the specified time frame (usually ten to fifteen days), an autopsy must be done to submit brain tissue to the appropriate state authorities for testing. The prognosis is *grave*.

All persons in contact with the infected dog may need to go through a series of post-exposure vaccines. State and county health departments oversee these procedures. Many veterinarians and animal health personnel get prophylactic pre-exposure vaccines.

Borreliosis (Lyme Disease)

Lyme disease was first reported in Lyme, Connecticut, in 1977. This disease originally was thought to affect only people. We have since learned it can affect most mammals. It is becoming very prevalent in the United States. Lyme disease has been reported in forty-seven states, concentrated in the northeast. Lyme disease is caused by the spirochete *Borrelia burgdorferi*, which is a corkscrew-shaped bacterium.

The natural host of the spirochete is the *Ixodes*, or deer tick. This tick lives outdoors in grassy and wooded areas. The adults normally attach and feed from wild animals, especially the white-tailed deer. The adults lay eggs outside in the spring. The eggs hatch, and the larvae begin their feeding, usually on any warm-blooded animal but most typically mice and other small rodents. They feed only once as larvae. They then molt into nymphs, which live for several months, feeding many times during that period. The nymphs are about the size of poppy seeds, and peak between May and July. Latest reports show that about 25 percent of nymph deer ticks carry Lyme disease. It generally takes twenty-four to forty-eight hours of feeding on the host for the tick to transmit the disease. By early autumn, the nymphs molt again into adults. Approximately 50 percent of the adult deer ticks now carry Lyme disease. Adults generally live for two years.

Exposure to the ticks occurs through brushing up against grass, shrubs, tree branches and other vegetation that harbors the insects. They literally wait for a warm-blooded creature to walk by, and they climb onto the animal or person. They are climbers, so they crawl upward toward the head where they "bite" or attach themselves to the skin. Therefore, staying out of the woods and grassy pastures dramatically cuts down on exposure. Check yourself and your pets for ticks after every jaunt in the woods. Since Lyme disease takes twenty-four to forty-eight hours to develop, pulling the ticks out shortly after attachment prevents infection.

Tick removal is not as tricky as most people think. We use rubbing alcohol to stun the tick first (provided it's not near the eyes) and splinter tweezers to remove it. Grasp the bug's head area as close to the skin as you can, and give a firm twist and pull. If the head of the tick is left in, don't make a surgical procedure to cut it out. It won't come easily since it is barbed like a fish hook; usually the heads work themselves out on their own like a small splinter would.

The mode of transmission is through the adults and nymph tick bites, as the newly hatched larvae do not yet carry the disease. The life cycle is described here:

> **Egg.** Eggs are laid by females in a single batch of thousands. This is done in the environment, not on the host. The eggs hatch into larvae in several weeks. The larvae then look for a host to feed on—usually the first warm-blooded animal that walks by.

> **Larva.** The larva hatches from the egg and finds a warm-blooded host. It could be a wild or domestic animal. It feeds once for several days, then drops off into the environment and molts into a nymph-stage tick. In tick-borne diseases, the larva doesn't carry the disease.

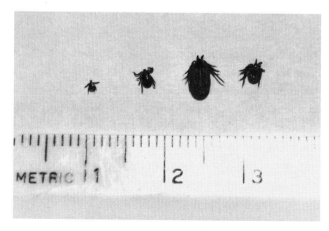

Deer ticks. From left to right, larva, nymph, adult female, and adult male.

Nymph. Ticks at this stage also need to feed on a warm-blooded host. After a few days of molting, the new nymph is ready to hitchhike a ride and grab a meal. After feeding for about a week, it drops off again to molt. This process can take months, but does produce an adult. In tick-borne diseases, the nymph can carry the disease.

Adult. As you can see, the adult tick is the result of a very lengthy process that involves several months, three moltings, and lots of cooperation from three different hosts! Adult ticks can live for nearly two years.

Use of insect repellents such as tick sprays, collars, dips and powders will discourage the tick from attaching itself to the pet. If the tick is persistent and stays, the insecticide will usually kill it within twenty-four to thirty-six hours. Not all tick products can be used on all pets; that is, some may be for either puppies or adult dogs only. Read all labels carefully, and always use as directed. A few new products are available to prevent tick bites. These come as either a tick collar with the active ingredient amitraz, or a permethrin oil, applied monthly.

Symptoms in animals are very similar to those in people. It can take weeks to months for an exposure to incubate into disease and symptoms. The classic "bull's eye" rash, often seen in people, is not reliable in animals, and most tick bites (whether Lyme disease is present or not) leave a raised lump for days at the site of attachment. Therefore, the most reliable indicator of disease is either clinical symptoms or a continually rising Lyme titer. Symptoms are fever, loss of appetite, swollen aching joints, general body aching and lameness. There is a loss of appetite due to the fever. The spirochete gets into the joints, where it stimulates an inflammatory reaction. There can be permanent damage to the joint surfaces, leading to chronic arthritis. Some puppies are hit so hard they seem almost paralyzed. If left untreated, Lyme disease can progress to life-threatening cardiac, neurologic or renal (kidney) failure. There have been reports of seizures and convulsions in Lyme-positive dogs. This spirochete can invade and destroy both heart muscle and kidney tissue. In our experience, the renal failure is more common. Once the disease destroys kidney tissue, the prognosis is *grave*.

Diagnosis is made by putting together the patient's history ("Our puppy is always in the woods") and a clinical presentation as described previously. A Lyme titer—which is a quantitative measure of the animal's immunity, or antibody level, to a particular disease—is also administered. One titer result, however, is not always enough to make a diagnosis. I like to run two or even three, if necessary, to follow a trend in the numbers.

There is some discussion as to the accuracy of these tests. Occasionally you get "false negatives," which means that the titer may come back negative in spite of Lyme being present in the animal's system. This is usually because there is a window of about four to six weeks after exposure when the titer is on its way up but is not into a positive range yet. Taking another test four weeks later will often reveal that the titer has risen into the positive range.

Another confusing factor is that many dogs who are seropositive (meaning they have a positive titer test) are not sick and show no symptoms—and may never.

Finally, there can be cross-reactivity of antibodies with other bacteria. This means that the titer blood test is not 100 percent specific to B. *burgdorferi*. These are called "false positives."

Therefore, the diagnosis of Lyme disease is made by considering both the clinical presentation of the dog as well as the ancillary blood tests. One recent advance is a titer test called the *western blot* test. It can differentiate between antibodies from an actual infection of Lyme disease and antibodies from the vaccine (described further on). This becomes very useful when testing a dog that received the *Borrelia* vaccine. Before this test, a positive result was hard to interpret; was the positive from Lyme disease or the vaccine?

Regardless of the means of making a diagnosis, once it has been reached, treatment is started. This usually involves long-term antibiotics (weeks to months). Progress is evaluated by monitoring the diminution of clinical signs and a falling titer. Of the two, the titer is the less reliable because the antibody levels can stay elevated for months following a natural infection. We find it more useful to follow trends in these titers. A downward trend implies that the immune system is no longer producing antibodies to the bacteria, which suggests it is clear of it.

There are two Lyme vaccines available through veterinarians. They are used as an adjunct to the other preventive measures described. The first one came out in July 1990. Our experience with it has been favorable. It is only for dogs, and annual boosters are required to keep up the protective immunity. A recent report found that the vaccine was more effective in dogs that had not yet been exposed to the disease (about 86 percent prevention) versus those that already showed a positive titer (about 58 percent prevention). This implies that puppies should be vaccinated young prior to any exposure for the vaccine to be more effective. The report found few post-vaccine reactions. Most were mild and were resolved without any treatment.

At time of printing, the second of the Lyme vaccines came on the market. This one is *bivalent*, which means that there are two strains of the *Borrelia* organism in it.

Common sense says the vaccine should be used in Lyme-endemic areas where there is a real threat of contracting the disease. Our protocol is to test each puppy's titer prior to vaccination. If the puppy is positive, we treat it first, recheck the titer in one month, then vaccinate if negative. The reason we don't vaccinate seropositive dogs is that there could be an immune-like reaction, causing symptons similar to Lyme disease.

Chapter 3

Parasites That Affect Your Puppy

his chapter is devoted to all the common "bugs" of puppies. We use the term loosely. We are really referring to the parasites of dogs. A parasite is an organism that lives on or in another living thing; in this case, your puppy. Some parasites live peacefully with their host; others do not, causing disease. Parasites are generally bugs, worms or protozoan microscopic organisms. We will not consider bacteria, fungi, or viruses as parasites. The chapter is divided into two groups, external and internal parasites, and provides information on the following:

- Which parasites invade dogs
- Where and how the parasite lives
- How your puppy got exposed to it
- What disease the parasite causes, and how serious the disease is
- Whether it is contagious to other animals or people
- How to get rid of the parasite

The good news is that most of these parasites are more of a nuisance than a real health concern. The exceptions will be noted as we go along. Some are contagious to people, so we will highlight those. Don't be surprised if you start finding yourself itch while you read about some of these bugs; some actually do get under your skin! There are many days when our staff at the clinic imagines we have bugs crawling on us after a long day of seeing fleas, ticks or mange. I have actually gone home after a particularly "buggy" day and used a flea shampoo on myself!

Common External Parasites

These bugs live on or in the skin of animals (and some live on people). Some you can see; others you can't. Some get into your house and make a home to breed in; others live entirely on the pet. All are crawling insects; none have wings or fly. And for those of you who think a bug is a bug is a bug, this chapter will change your mind.

Ear Mites. The scientific name for these small bugs that live in dogs' ear canals is *Otodectes*. This bug is a mite, which is a microscopic bug that feeds on the outer layers of the skin (epidermis). Mites live for two months and have a three-week life cycle, the time it takes to develop from an egg into an adult. They inhabit the surface of the ear canal and do not burrow in the skin. Your veterinarian can see them with the use of the otoscope (a fancy flashlight that has a magnifying glass and a long nose to see deep into the ear canal). You can actually see many of them crawling around.

Symptoms are intense itching of the ears, shaking of the head, constant scratching of the ears, a dark brown waxy discharge that looks like "coffee grounds" and crusting and flaking of the upper ear canal. Occasionally, the incessant scratching may cause bleeding of the outer ear.

Treatment consists of a thorough cleaning of the ear canals with a ceruminolytic agent (a wash that loosens wax). Since most of the waxy debris is deep in the ear canal, cleaning usually means flushing it out. This should be done by a veterinarian. If it is done too vigorously, you run the risk of rupturing the tympanum (or eardrum). Once the ears are clean, an ear mite preparation is put into the ear. These are drops that contain an insecticide and a soap. Many brands are available, but the better ones only require one or two applications a week for two weeks. There is evidence that the mites can briefly come out of the ear and crawl on the dog's fur. If this is suspected, the dog should be treated with an insecticide dip, spray or powder (these are flea and tick products). The presence of mites should be verified before treatment for them begins, as this disease mimics other types of ear infections.

It is generally thought that these mites don't inhabit houses or infect people. There is a report, however, which documents that under certain conditions these mites can live in the house and cause an allergy in people similar to that caused by house mites. Therefore, we will consider ear mites a minor human health hazard.

Lice (Pediculosis). We see lice on puppies that come from shelters, kennels, pet stores or any situation where crowding occurs. Lice are small insects measuring only two millimeters in length that live on the hair shafts. They literally cling to the hair with their claws. They spend

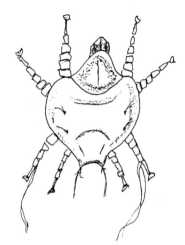

Drawing of an ear mite (Otodectes).

their entire life cycle on the host; they cannot live off the host. They feed by either eating the flaking outer layer of skin (epidermis) or sucking blood. Lice are contagious among dogs. Physical contact is needed to transfer lice from one dog to another. Lice lay their eggs (called *nits*) attached to hair shafts. These eggs are firmly cemented to the hair shaft and look like small white dots. You need a special comb to remove them. Visual inspection of the eggs is easier with a magnifying glass. Some vets use transparent tape pressed to the fur to harvest some of the bugs and eggs for microscopic examination. This is called the "tape test."

Symptoms are intense itching and scratching, with hair loss. If the infestation is heavy, an anemia can occur due to blood loss (caused by the bloodsucking type of lice). These signs can be mistaken for other skin diseases. Your veterinarian can differentiate among these similar but different diseases.

Treatment is fairly easy. Most of the products made to kill fleas and ticks also kill lice. The active ingredient, pyrethrin, is well-suited for this. If the dog has mats of hair, it should be shaved prior to use of shampoos or dips. All grooming tools should be washed in a pyrethrin-based solution to kill any lice that linger. All other dogs that have come into contact with the patient should be tested for lice. Any dog suffering from anemia should be treated with iron supplements.

Lice are very host-specific and do not cross species. This means that human lice stay on people and dog lice stay on dogs. Dog lice are not contagious to people, and vice versa.

Mange Mites

Mange mites are similar to the ear mites described previously. The difference is that mange mites live everywhere but in the ears. Each of the three distinct manges described are very different in some aspects, but similar in others. We will give you an idea of how they are similar and how they differ. To start off with, let's look at the similarities. All three are caused by mange mites. All three live in or on the skin. All three are common in young puppies. All three cause intense itching and skin disease. And all three are diagnosed the same way. Where they differ is in the prognosis, severity and treatment, and the health hazards they pose to humans. Each of them is described in detail in this section.

Cheyletiella or "Walking Dandruff." This mange is caused by the cheyletiella mite. These mites live on the surface of the skin. They crawl and creep along the back spine, leaving a bad case of dandruff in their wake. These mites are large in comparison to other mites, but you still can't see them with the naked eye. They are not as host-specific as lice: They can be shared among dogs, cats, rabbits and, occasionally, people. They don't suck blood, but they do live off the fluids of the skin. They spend their entire life on the dog and cannot live off their host. They do not inhabit the house.

The most noticeable symptom is an intensely itchy case of dandruff along the back of the dog. The dandruff is so severe it should really be called seborrhea. Regular shampooing will not control it. Simply put, this is an itchy dandruff that won't quit.

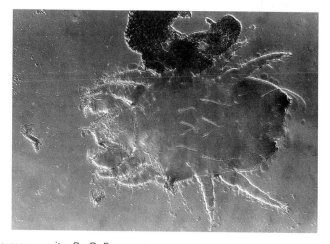

Cheyletiella mange mite. *Dr. D. Bowman.*

Diagnosis is made by one of three different methods: 1) examination of the fur with a magnifying glass, 2) use of transparent tape pressed to the fur to lift mites off to be studied under a microscope, or 3) use of a skin scraping, a description of which follows:

Step 1: The veterinarian wets a scalpel blade with mineral oil.

Step 2: The scalpel blade is scraped on the surface of the affected skin to harvest loose crusts and scabs onto the blade. This is done with moderate pressure.

Step 3: The skin debris on the blade is scraped off onto a clean glass microscope slide.

Step 4: The slide is inspected under the microscope for identification of the mites.

Once the diagnosis of cheyletiella is made, treatment is started immediately. These bugs are very easy to kill with pyrethrin flea and tick preparations. Shampooing with a pyrethrin shampoo followed by a complete cleaning or fumigation of the dog's bedding and sleeping quarters is essential. This procedure should be continued weekly for two to three weeks. Powders and sprays work well too, but are messy.

The cheyletiella mite can infect people. Breeders who have a litter of puppies afflicted with the mite often report getting very itchy red bites that drain fluid and leave a yellow-crusted lesion. These infections are usually self-limiting and may resolve in three to four weeks. People who suspect that they have this condition should consult a dermatologist for treatment options.

Demodectic Mange. This mange is caused by the demodex mite, a cigar-shaped mite that lives in the hair follicles. A small number of these mites normally live in a dog's skin. When they overpopulate, however, they cause a severe dermatitis. These mites are transferred by the dam (mother) to the puppies shortly after birth via nursing. In a healthy puppy, these mites are kept to low numbers by a normally functioning immune system. Puppies that are stressed, malnourished, burdened with parasites, underweight, sick with other illness or immunosuppressed are more likely to get this mange. Demodetic mange is not contagious to people and is barely contagious to other normal adult dogs. Luckily, these bugs cannot live off the host, so they don't infect the house. There are two forms of demodectic mange: localized and generalized.

Localized Demodex. As the name implies, localized demodex means the mange is confined to a small area, usually around the face, head and legs. These areas are patches of itchy, bald, red, raised skin. The most common areas are on the muzzle and around the eyes. The lesions often start at three months of age. Diagnosis is made by the veterinarian performing a skin scraping.

Treatment of a localized lesion usually involves daily application of a Rotenone ointment to the lesion. The interesting thing is that if no treatment is done, most of these cases resolve on their own as the puppy's immune system matures, usually by six months. The prognosis is *fair* to *good*. These puppies rarely go on to develop generalized lesions.

Generalized Demodex. This form is much more widespread on the body, covering large patches of the head and neck, chest, flank and abdomen. It may start as localized but quickly spread to other parts of the body. The diagnosis is made using the skin-scraping technique described previously. The inflammatory response is so severe that the dog may run a fever and have enlarged lymph nodes. There is often secondary bacterial infection with *Staphylococcus* bacteria. The overpopulation of mites grows out of the hair follicle and into the surrounding dermis (deeper layer of the skin). This in turn causes abscesses in the dermis we call *deep pyoderma* or *furunculosis.* At this point, the disease is life-threatening and carries a *poor* prognosis.

This form is much more difficult to treat. Up to 50 percent of the body may be involved. It is impractical to smear ointment over this large an area. In these cases we use dips, or drenches, to cover the entire dog. Dips are most effective when the dog's skin is stripped of crusts and matted fur. This must be done by a veterinarian, and not a groomer, as this dip is a strong chemical. The dip is done every other week for three to four treatments. One report found an 86 percent success rate with this protocol. Due to the secondary bacterial infection, the use of antibiotics formulated for skin usage (meaning they will kill *Staphylococcus*) may be needed. Some veterinarians are tempted to use strong anti-inflammatory drugs, such as cortisone, to relieve the itch and pain. This should be avoided at all cost, as the cortisone will lower the dog's already faltering immune system and make matters worse.

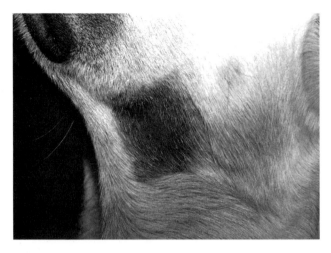

Localized demodex appears as patches of itchy, bald skin, usually around the face. head and legs.

There is a predisposition in short-coated breeds for generalized demodex.

Sarcoptic Mange. The other name for this mange is *scabies*. The mite is *Sarcoptes scabiei*. These mites look like little crabs under the microscope. They live by burrowing into the upper layers of the skin, where they lay their eggs and make tunnels. These mites live deeper in the skin than the Cheyletiella mite. Their life cycle is three weeks. The areas of the body most often affected are the legs, tail, underside of abdomen and head. This condition has been described as one in which the dog gets "eaten alive from the ground up."

Symptoms are an inexhaustible, intense itch that spreads. The skin becomes inflamed, red and crusty; and the hair falls out. The itch is incessant, so the dog invariably scratches constantly, which leads to open sores and secondary bacterial infection. To watch this process, one would think the dog is literally being consumed by something. A wrong diagnosis can lead to a terrible mistake: If an allergy is suspected and the vet administers cortisone, the disease can worsen suddenly. A veterinarian who has seen this enough will come to recognize a certain odor from the skin. In our clinic, we say the dog smells "mangy." Diagnosis is made by the veterinarian performing a skin scraping, as described in the section on Cheyletiella.

The elusive nature of this mite makes it particularly difficult to diagnose. One report states that mites are found in only 50 percent of

The Mange Mites

Mite Name	Where It Lives on Skin	Symptoms	Where on Body Signs Appear	Diagnosis	Treatment	Human Hazard
Cheyletiella	Surface	Excess Flaking	Along Back	Skin Scraping	Pyrethrin Dips	YES
Demodectic	Hair Follicle	Itching, Bald Spots	Face, Head and Legs	Skin Scraping	Goodwinol or Mitaban Dips	NO
Sarcoptic	Deeper Skin in Tunnels	Intense Itch, Yellow Crusts	Legs, Head and Underside	Skin Scraping	Lime-Sulfur Dip, Ivermectin Injection	YES

the cases. If a veterinarian even suspects the existence of this disease, he or she should start treatment even if mites have not actually been found in a skin scraping.

Treatment used to be dips of a horribly smelly lime-sulfur shampoo that smells like rotten eggs and can stink up an entire clinic for a day or two. We can't imagine the dog enjoyed it any more. These dips were given weekly for four to six times, which became costly for the owner. Now the treatment of choice is two injections two weeks apart of the ivermectin anthelmintic. Although this drug is not yet approved by the FDA for this purpose, it is widely used in small-animal medicine, as well as in laboratory animals. It is effective for most mange. This drug should not be used in Collies or Shetland Sheepdogs, due to a sensitivity to the drug. These breeds will have to rely on the lime-sulfur shampoos.

This mange is contagious to people. Luckily, these bugs cannot live off the host, so they don't infect the house. Anyone who is in physical contact with the patient is at risk of getting it. The bites look like small red dots that itch. These progress to a yellow crust. Generally, sarcoptic mange mites don't like human hosts (we don't have enough hair for them). Most human cases spontaneously resolve without treatment within four weeks of the dog being treated. If you notice symptoms similar to these on yourself, we recommend you consult your dermatologist.

Fleas

The scientific name for this bug is *Ctenocephalides*. All of us know how annoying fleas are. They have been a nuisance to man for millenia. The Egyptians were plagued with them and wrote about how to exterminate them in

1555 B.C. It was common, through the nineteenth century, for people in all socioeconomic classes throughout much of the world to be infested with fleas (though they were different fleas than the ones that infest animals).

All fleas can be easily seen with the naked eye. They're about the size of sesame seeds. They are brownish-red in color and run very fast. When off the dog, they can jump six feet in one hop. Your puppy picked them up by either going outside in a grassy area, or from another dog or cat that had them. Fleas have four stages in their thirty-day life cycle: the egg, larva, pupa and adult, as described next.

Egg. The egg is white, oval and glossy. You can see the eggs with a magnifying glass. One female can lay hundreds of eggs in her life. Most are laid on the pet, then fall off into the house—especially where the dog sleeps. The eggs will hatch in a couple of weeks under the right temperature and humidity conditions (warm and humid).

Larva. The larvae are what emerge from the eggs. They look like small worms and can be seen with a magnifying glass. The larvae stay in the rug or bedding, or go under furniture where it's dark. They molt several times over a period of weeks to months. The final stage of the larva spins a cocoon and is then called a pupa. These cocoons are usually found in carpet fibers or under furniture.

Pupa. These insects are undergoing changes in the cocoon, turning into adult fleas. This process is quite variable and can take weeks to months. Vibration of the floor can stimulate the adult to hatch out of the cocoon and look for a host. Many of us who inadvertently leave for vacation with flea eggs in the house know all too well how just the vibration of the door closing and you walking around when you return

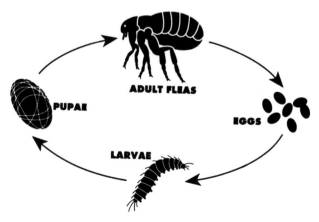

The flea life cycle.

stimulates all the pupae to hatch. Within minutes, your ankles are covered in newly hatched, hungry adult fleas!

Adult. The adults are what most of us see on the dog. They bite and suck blood. They are like heat-seeking missiles, targeting any warm body. Their feces are the black specks we call "flea dirt." If owners don't actually see the adults, they usually see the black specks and comment, "It looks like someone sprinkled ground black peppercorns on my dog!" The adults are the only form that bite the dog. Adult fleas can live for over a month under the right conditions. The flea saliva is very irritating to most dogs, which starts an allergic reaction. The dog develops red swellings and intense itching at the bite site. This causes the common biting and scratching the owners report. The dog may have such a violent reaction as to cause self-mutilation, hair loss and a secondary bacterial infection. We call this *flea allergy dermatitis* (FAD).

As you can see from this life cycle, fleas can reproduce very quickly. In fact, several adults can multiply into a couple of thousand in one month! Your pets, house and sometimes family members all become infected with these blood-sucking bugs. The places where fleas are commonly found on a dog are the lower back near the base of tail, between the legs, the underside of the abdomen and the inner thighs. Occasionally they will wander to other areas, but they don't stay long. The common site for flea bites on people is the ankle.

Not only do these bugs cause itching and allergic dermatitis, but they can carry disease. The dog flea can carry the tapeworm *Dipylidium caninum*. Therefore, any puppy infested with fleas should be either tested or treated for tapeworms (more later on tapeworms in this chapter).

Treatment for fleas is twofold: it involves treating the dog and its environment. The reason is that treating only one will not break the life cycle, leading to an uninterrupted breeding cycle. People who treat either the dog or the house only will never get rid of their flea problem.

Treating the Dog

The first thing most people do when they see fleas is give their dog a flea bath. This is fine for killing the adult fleas on the dog, but as already discussed, this is only part of the problem. What about the eggs and larvae on the dog? What about the eggs and larvae in the house? What about the adults in the house? For now, let's concentrate on the pet. As you can imagine, you will be limited to using products approved for use on dogs. Most products have a minimum age requirement. Generally speaking, the stronger the active ingredient, the older the puppy has to be. So many brands are out there that there isn't enough room here to cover them all. What we will do is review the most common active ingredients. This information is relevant regardless of the brand.

High-potency active ingredients: Carbamates (carbaryl), organophosphates (chlorpyrifos, cythioate, diazanon, dichlorvos, fenvalerate, fenthion, methylcarbamate, butoxypropylene, piperonyl butoxide, malathion) and rotenone.

- These should not be used in puppies under sixteen weeks old and should be used with caution in older puppies.
- They have the potential for toxic side effects, such as excess salivation, dilated pupils, muscle twitching, vomiting and diarrhea. Toxicity has led to death in some cases.
- Side effects should be treated promptly by a veterinarian.
- They are very effective.
- They kill adults only (except for chlorpyrifos, which can kill larvae).

Moderate-potency active ingredients: Pyrethrin, microencapsulated pyrethrin, allethrin, synergized pyrethroids and permethrin.

- Some preparations can be used in puppies as young as eight weeks old.
- There are mild and few side effects, which often resolve when the product is washed off the pet.
- They are very effective and generally safer than organophosphates, carbamates or rotenone.
- Some insect resistance occurs.
- Frequent applications may be necessary due to instability under bright light (less so for the microencapsulated and pyrethroid forms).
- They kill adults only.

Mildest-potency active ingredients: Orange peel derivatives (D-limonene, linalool).

- These can be used on puppies as young as six weeks of age.
- There are mild and few side effects.
- Their efficacy is modest; prolonged contact with the flea is needed to kill it.
- More resistance is seen.
- They kill adults only.

Topical Insect Growth Regulators: Methoprene, fenoxycarb.

- They prevent the normal progression of the flea's life cycle. In effect, they prevent the egg and/or larva from becoming an adult. Since most of the female fleas lay eggs on the dog, if the egg came into contact with a growth regulator prior to falling off, it would not develop or hatch in the house.
- They are safe for puppies as young as eight weeks old.
- They are safe and effective alternatives or adjuncts to insecticides, and are used worldwide in drinking water to reduce the mosquito population.
- They are used very effectively in combination with an adulticide for controlling recurrent flea infestations.
- To see any insect resistance is unusual.

Home Remedies: Brewer's yeast, garlic cloves, menthol, eucalyptus, citronella, herbal extracts.

- These products are more repellents than insecticides.
- Many people swear by these, although there is little scientific evidence that they work.
- No toxicity occurs; most are either food additives or botanicals.
- They can be used on young puppies six weeks old.

All these active ingredients come in a variety of forms: shampoos, sprays, powders, collars, dips, pouches of oil and mousse foam. Each vet or groomer has a personal preference as to which are best. Each is briefly described next:

Shampoo. These are just like shampoos you'd use on yourself. The dog is wet, then lathered with the shampoo. It is important to leave the shampoo on the dog for ten minutes to ensure it works. Always start lathering on the head and work your way down to the tail. Be careful not to get any in the eyes. A thorough rinsing is needed to wash out any soap residue. Remember, once the shampoo is rinsed off, there is no residual activity. This means the dog has no protection left.

Sprays. These are liquids that contain insecticides which are sprayed directly on the dog. They may have a water or alcohol base. Most of them dry quickly and have a strong chemical odor. Each one is different, and directions must be followed closely. Sprays usually have a lasting effect of several days. This means that they must be reapplied regularly.

Powders. These are body powders that contain an insecticide. These are messy, and many people object to the "cloud" that surrounds the dog when it walks. Many dogs are allergic to these and will sneeze for days after the application. Powders need to be reapplied regularly.

Collars. These are neck collars that release an insecticide over time. Collars work best in small breeds, where there isn't as much distance between the collar and the base of the tail, where fleas like to live. These have a definite life span, usually several months. The biggest fault people have is forgetting how old the collar is and letting it expire. Collars seem to work best when used with other flea products.

Dips. These are strong concentrates that are mixed with water and sponged onto the dog, but not rinsed. Another name for these is "drench." When they dry, a fine residual powder is left on the fur and usually lasts from two to four weeks. If you use a dip, you should not use any other insecticide products with it for fear of overdosing your dog and causing a toxicity. Many veterinarians and groomers routinely use dips. Be advised: Very young, old or sick dogs should not have dips.

Oil Pouches. These are small pouches of permethrin oil that are applied to the skin on the dog's back. The fine oil spreads evenly over the dog's body and remains on the skin for up to one month if not washed off. According to the manufacturer, the oil is not absorbed through the skin.

Mousse. This is a foam spray that has an insecticide as its active ingredient. It is particularly useful when you cannot wet the animal's coat. We use it on the face, where other products may be awkward (especially near the eyes).

Other products are available, from electronic collars to oral tablets where the insecticide gets into the dog's bloodstream and kills the flea when it bites. Our concern with the tablets is that they introduce a continual serum blood level of organophosphates in a young developing puppy. We do not recommend these products under normal circumstances, although we concede their merit under certain conditions—for example, in southern states, where flea problems are year-round.

Oral insect growth inhibitors: A recent addition to the family of flea products is a once-a-month pill you give to your dog that causes the flea to become sterile when it bites your dog. It contains an insect development inhibitor that is safe for mammals, but prevents the female flea's eggs from developing normally, breaking the flea life cycle. I consider this more flea control for the home, because it doesn't prevent fleas from living on and biting your puppy. But at least they won't be able to infest your house, which anyone who has ever had fleas in the house will agree!

Top Ten Guidelines for Flea Product Usage

1. Always follow the label directions on all flea products. Don't assume one product is like another.

2. Be careful to use products that are FDA-approved for use in puppies. Most labels will list the minimum age for which the product is safe.

3. Use the product only as frequently as the label says. If it says to apply once weekly, then do so.

4. Follow all the label warning instructions. Some products require the administrator to wear gloves or eye protection. Also, almost all the products have child hazard warnings. Be careful, and follow all warnings.

5. Treat all the animals in the house on the same day. Unfortunately, staggering the animals won't work.

6. If you like to see a "quick kill" of the adult fleas, shampoos and dips work the best. It's so rewarding to see the little bugs wash down the drain.

7. If your puppy won't cooperate for a bath, then sprays are your answer because they don't require you to soak the animal with anything. Usually a gentle misting over the entire animal (except the face) is all that's needed. Rub the spray into the dog's coat afterward. This gets the spray down to skin level where the fleas live.

8. We consider powders, collars and mousses to be adjuncts to the previously mentioned techniques.

9. Permethrin oil pouches have been very effective, easy to apply and long-lasting. They kill both fleas and ticks, and can be used with other products. Unfortunately, they are not for use on puppies under six months of age. A drawback is that they can leave the coat a little greasy.

10. We recommend the use of insect growth regulators whenever possible to break the reproductive cycle of the adult fleas.

Treating the House

As described in the previous section, many products are available to kill fleas. The products designed for the premises, or house, are not to be used on the dog. This might be confusing at first, especially when you see that the active ingredients are the same as those in the dog products. The difference is usually in their concentrations. The premise sprays contain active ingredients in too high a concentration to be safely used on pets. *Please refer to the preceding descriptions of the products for further information on active ingredients.*

Fewer products are available for treating the house than for treating the dog (no dips or mousse can be used for the house). The better products contain active ingredients to kill adult fleas, as well as insect growth regulators. They also boast long (up to one year) residuals. Most of these products are for people to treat their own homes. The alternative is to have your home professionally treated by an exterminator.

Following are the different forms of insecticide products for the premises:

Powders. These are dusting powders that contain a variety of active ingredients to kill adult fleas. The product needs to be dusted over most of the floor, including under furniture. Carpets are targeted more than hardwood or tiled floors. These tend to be messy, and most owners vacuum up the powder due to the mess. People with allergies should be especially careful while using these products. Always follow the manufacturer's directions.

Sprays. These come as either pump sprays or pressurized aerosols. They contain a variety of active ingredients to kill adult as well as pre-adult fleas. Long residuals are common. These are much less messy than powders, but there are fumes and a strong odor from most of them. People with allergies should be especially careful while using these products. Always follow the manufacturer's directions.

Foggers. These are cans of pressured insecticide that are set off in specific rooms. They spew out a fog of insecticide that fumigates every nook and cranny. They are highly effective and usually contain adulticide as well as insect growth regulators. The drawbacks are that the house has to be vacated during the process, then aired out; and birds, aquariums and some plants need to be removed from the house. As you can see, this process is more involved. People with allergies should be especially careful while using these products. Always follow the manufacturer's directions.

Guidelines for House Treatment

1. Always follow the label directions on all flea products. Don't assume one product is like another.

2. Be careful to use products that are FDA-approved for use in homes. Most labels will list the appropriate surfaces the product is safe to use on (drapes, upholstery, wood floors, rugs, etc.).

3. Use the product only as frequently as the label says.

4. Follow all the label warning instructions. Some products require the administrator to wear gloves or eye protection. Also, almost all these products have child hazard warnings. Be careful, and follow all warnings.

5. *All* rooms the dog goes in should be treated.

6. Start by vacuuming all the flooring and carpets in the house. This means under furniture and baseboards. Throw out the vacuum bag afterwards so that you're not harboring fleas in your vacuum.

7. Launder all pet bedding. This is a favorite place for fleas to live and eggs to hatch. If laundering is not possible, throw the bedding out.

8. Remove all small items from the room, like plants, baskets, towel racks, pillows, etc. The fewer items there are, the better the product can infiltrate.

9. Try to use products that contain both an adulticide and an insect growth regulator. You want to kill both the adults and eggs! Otherwise, you'll need to do this all over again in three to four weeks.

10. The best time to do this is when the pets, adults and kids are out of the house. The pets should be treated for fleas at the same time, either outside or at your local veterinarian's office or groomer's.

11. Leave enough time for this procedure. It doesn't pay to rush it. Remember, haste makes waste. If you forget a step or don't cover the entire area, you'll be doing it all over again.

12. Your veterinarian will be most happy to help you with your flea problem, so ask lots of questions. He or she probably has their own system for flea control, including the necessary products. They are professionals in flea control.

Most people find exterminating fleas a major headache. The process can be very involved if there are multiple pets or a large living space to treat. We can tell you with certainty that if you don't follow the appropriate steps in a timely fashion, you will not get rid of your flea problem. If nothing works for you, hire a professional exterminator.

The most common reasons for failure in treating your flea problem are the following:

- Treatment of the pets was not done *at the same time* as the treatment of the house.
- Treatment of *all furry pets* in the house, especially cats, was not done *at the same time*.
- Ineffective products were used, perhaps due to resistance of the flea to the active ingredient.
- Not enough product was used to effectively kill the fleas. *Follow directions!*
- Furniture was not moved when applying a product for the house. You must get under all furniture.
- When treating the dog, you did not get into every crevice of the animal (except eyes). This means between toes, behind ears, under tail and between legs. These are some of the fleas' favorite hiding places.
- A product was used that didn't contain an insect growth regulator, so only adults were killed. Any eggs in the rug and floor crevices are still going to hatch.
- The product was outdated. Check for expiration dates.
- You forgot to throw away the vacuum bag after vacuuming for fleas. In effect, you made a flea hotel in your vacuum.

Ticks

Ticks are small, wingless insects that normally live outdoors. They vary in size from a poppy seed to a large grape, depending on the stage, species and state of engorgement (how much blood they've consumed). They are true parasites in that they feed by sucking blood from the host. They come in two varieties: hard and soft. The ticks that parasitize dogs are hard. This means that there is a shield (called a *scutum*) to protect the body. The tick life cycle has four stages:

Egg. They are laid by females in a single batch of thousands. This is done in the environment, not on the host. The eggs hatch into larvae in several weeks. The larvae then look for a host to feed on, usually the first warm-blooded animal that walks by.

Larva. The larva hatches from the egg and finds a warm-blooded host. It could be a wild or domestic animal. It feeds for several days, then drops off into the environment and molts into a nymph-stage tick. In tick-borne diseases, the larvae don't carry the disease.

Nymph. Ticks at this stage also need to feed on a warm-blooded host. After a few days of molting, the new nymph is ready to hitchhike a ride and grab a meal. After feeding for about a week, it drops off again to molt. This process can take months, but does produce an adult.

Adult. As you can see, the adult tick is the result of a very lengthy process that involves months, three moltings, and lots of cooperation from three different hosts! Adult ticks can live for nearly two years. They carry tick-borne diseases, like Rocky Mountain spotted fever and Lyme disease.

Ticks are often found in certain locales, or in pockets. One neighborhood may be crawling with them, while the adjacent area may be devoid of them. Why? These insects thrive in certain environmental conditions—namely, damp and shady areas. Sunny pastures or dry land may not be able to sustain their life cycle. Wooded, grassy and thickly settled areas with shrubs are perfect places to find ticks.

Ticks are natural climbers. This means that once on a dog, they climb upward until they reach the head and neck (unless they get lost on the way, which sometimes happens). This explains why most ticks are found on the head, especially the ears.

Once the tick settles into a comfortable spot, it "bites" the dog. This involves inserting its barbed long nose (called a *capitulum*) into the dog's skin to feed. The barbs make the apparatus look much like a fishhook. This makes removing these tenacious little bugs very difficult.

Removing a Tick

All dog owners are faced with removing a tick from their dog from time to time, unless the dog never leaves its urban home. The technique we use in the clinic is to "stun" the tick with rubbing alcohol (unless it's near the eyes, in which case we use mineral oil). This means soaking a cotton swab with rubbing alcohol and placing it on the tick for thirty to sixty seconds. This disrupts the tick and often causes it to start backing out of the dog. But remember those barbs. These ticks don't just let go. They need to be pulled out, which takes some force. Grasp the head of the tick as close to the skin as

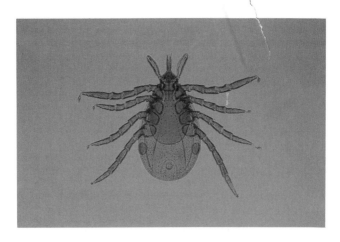

An adult deer tick, magnified many times. *Dr. D. Bowman*

possible. You may need to use tweezers for this. Give a quick twist and pull to remove the tick. What can often happen is that you break off the capitulum, leaving it in the skin. We call this "leaving the head in." But don't worry. The small black spot is like a splinter and usually works itself out on its own. Remember: Because of the barbs, you can't just pull the tick out like a splinter. You'd actually have to cut it out to remove it. Most vets and dog owners don't go through all that for a tick. And despite popular belief, the head does *not* grow into a new tick. The remaining bump left from the tick bite should be cleaned with a topical antiseptic, and an antibiotic ointment should be applied twice daily for a week to prevent infection. Try not to over-handle the tick so that doesn't break in your hand. Ticks can carry certain diseases that you wouldn't want to get on your hands.

Guidelines for Tick Prevention

The best way to prevent tick bites is to keep your puppy inside. This is impractical for most of us outdoor-loving people. But you can keep dogs out of heavily wooded areas and tall grassy fields. Here are some other tips:

- Avoid wooded areas and fields where you think wild animals live.
- Use a tick/insect repellent prior to taking your puppy outdoors. You may even want to use one on yourself.
- Wear light-colored clothes so that you can easily see any ticks that get on them. Wear white socks, and tuck your pants into them. Remember, ticks grab onto your legs as you and your puppy walk by.
- Inspect yourself and your puppy after each walk. Since the tick hasn't had time to bite yet, you'll find it crawling on the surface of the coat toward the head.

Tick Products

Most of the information regarding flea products pertains to ticks. But not all. You must read labels. If a product is approved by the FDA for ticks, it will say so on the label. Most products have a minimum age requirement. Generally speaking, the stronger the active ingredient, the older the puppy has to be. See the sections "Treating the Dog" and "Treating the House" for descriptions of each.

Diseases Ticks Carry

Ticks can be vectors (carriers) of disease. Not all diseases are found in all areas of the country. Following is a list of the three common tick-borne diseases in the U.S., with a brief description:

Rocky Mountain Spotted Fever (RMSF). This is a rickettsial disease cased by the *Rickettsia rickettsii* organism. The tick vector (carrier of disease) is the *Dermacentor* tick. Only certain areas of the US have this disease, most notably the southeast, although cases have been reported as far north as Long Island, New York. When a dog is bitten by a tick that carries RMSF, the symptoms ensue within two weeks. The organism causes a disturbance in blood clotting, leading to internal and subcutaneous (under the skin) bleeding. A rash develops, along with fever, vomiting and diarrhea, bloody urine and feces, nosebleeds and respiratory difficulty. Neurological signs such as seizures have been reported. A diagnosis is made by observing the clinical signs, finding a low platelet count on a complete blood count, and seeing a high positive result on the RMSF titer blood test. Treatment generally consists of several weeks of antibiotics, usually of the tetracycline family. The prognosis is *fair* to *good* if the disease is diagnosed and treated promptly.

Canine Ehrlichiosis. This is another tick-borne disease. Like Rocky Mountain spotted fever, the organism in ehrlichiosis is a rickettsial organism, namely *Ehrlichia canis*. The tick vector (carrier of disease) is a *Rhipicephalus* tick although some recent reports state that the deer tick is, too. The affected dogs develop a severe anemia, fever, bruising, edema of the extremities, and bleeding disorders. The white blood cells of these dogs are invaded by the organism and are rendered defective. There is a profound deficiency of *thrombocytes* (platelet cells responsible for blood clotting), which leads to excessive bleeding, as well as anemia and a low white blood cell count. The invading organism is often seen by the veterinarian on a blood smear.

The white blood cells can be concentrated for observation by a *buffy* coat procedure, in which the white blood cells are spun down by a centrifuge and harvested. They can then be smeared onto a slide for staining and microscopic exam.

Diagnosis is made by finding the organism on a blood smear, reduced levels of serum proteins and a high titer to the *ehrlichia* organism, as well as anemia and reduced white blood cell count. These dogs can either be in an acute phase, where there is much disease, or in a chronic state, where there is a slow insidious progression. Treatment is the administration of tetracycline or doxycycline antibiotics for several weeks. The prognosis is *fair* to *guarded*, depending on which phase the dog is in. The more chronic the case, the worse the prognosis.

Canine Babesiosis. This disease is also called *Piroplasmosis*. It has worldwide distribution and is very prominent in pockets throughout Europe. The organism is a protozoan called *Babesia* that invades red blood cells, causing a profound anemia and red blood cell destruction. The ticks of the *Dermacentor* and *Rhipicephalus* genera carry the protozoan.

The symptoms are fever, anemia, pale mucous membranes and a yellowing of the skin (jaundice). The spleen becomes enlarged and swollen from trapping all the infected, defective red blood cells. The jaundice is from the destruction of the red blood cells. The diagnosis is made from identifying the parasite on blood smears microscopically. There is also a titer test to measure the antibody levels to the organism. Treatment consists of anti-protozoan drugs. The prognosis is generally *fair* to *good*.

Borreliosis (Lyme Disease). There is a complete description of borreliosis in Chapter 2, under "Vaccine Diseases."

Common Internal Parasites

Unlike external parasites, the internal ones can cause severe disease and even death if left untreated. Imagine dozens of spaghetti-sized worms clogging up your heart valves, as is the case in canine heartworm disease. You can see how dangerous some of these internal parasites can be. Puppies are particularly susceptible to internal parasitism. In fact, many of the intestinal worms of puppies are transferred from the mother.

Roundworms (Ascariasis)

Roundworms belong to a group of parasites called *nematodes*, a group of worm-like parasites that affect most mammals. They live inside the host and measure from four to twenty centimeters in length. There are males and females that lay eggs and whose larvae go through four different molting phases to reach the adult. Each larva has a specific place it lives in the body. Most are migratory, which means they don't stay in one place very long. The adult worms settle in the small intestine, where they feed on the ingested food, robbing the host of nutrition. The roundworms that infect dogs are of the genus *Toxocara* or *Toxascaris*. Other genus can infect swine, horses, cattle, cats and wild animals. Let's look at the complicated life cycle of the dog roundworm.

Adults lay eggs in the intestines. Newly hatched larvae burrow through the intestinal wall and enter the bloodstream that goes to the liver. The larvae wander through the liver, then enter the bloodstream that flows through the heart and pulmonary arteries to enter the lungs. Larvae then migrate through the bronchi and are coughed up the trachea. Once coughed up, they are swallowed and complete their development in the stomach and small intestines, where the cycle starts all over again.

Just imagine the havoc and damage done from several dozen of these migrating larvae. It's a wake of destruction, so to speak. And this isn't the end of the story. Nature has it that in pregnant bitches, some of the larvae make their way to the placenta where they affect the developing fetuses. They also invade the mammary tissue and are passed on to the suckling pups. In this way, these worms can infect a litter of puppies either in utero (in the uterus) or by shedding larvae in the milk of the bitch.

What many breeders find frustrating is that adult dogs can harbor these larvae in their tissues for years. They can be very difficult to exterminate because these larvae are mostly resistant to the drugs we use to worm dogs. Therefore, litter after litter, a bitch can whelp puppies with roundworms

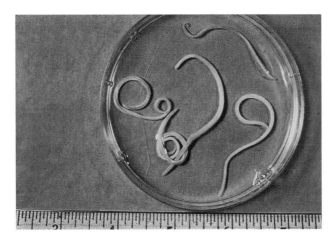

Adult Roundworms. *Dr. D. Bowman*

even though the bitch was wormed several times with the standard worming drugs. Another factor that propagates the worm burden is the fact that bitches usually lick up the puppy's feces (a cleaning instinct) in a whelping crate. Since most of the puppies are born with worms or get them shortly afterwards through the milk, the dam is reinfecting herself. Research is working on a wormer that will kill the larvae as well as the adult worms.

The symptoms of a roundworm infestation in a puppy are the following:

- Abdominal bloating
- Excess gas production
- Foul-smelling, loose diarrhea
- Bloody stools
- Emaciated puppies
- A chronic cough
- A poor, dry coat
- An insatiable appetite
- The passing of adult worms in vomit or feces
- Chronic poor-doer
- Anterior uveitis (inflammation of the inside eye)

The diagnosis of roundworms is made by either of two means: The puppy vomits up or passes adult roundworms in the stool, or the veterinarian performs a fecal exam (called a fecal flotation exam), which visualizes roundworm eggs under microscopic inspection.

Control of Roundworms. The most common wormers used to kill roundworms are piperazine and pyrantel pamoate. These drugs are given orally. They kill only the mature adult worms, so two wormings are needed three weeks apart (that's how long it takes larvae to become adults) to rid a puppy of a worm burden as described in this chart:

First Worming ⇩		**Second Worming** ⇩	
week 1	**week 2**		**week 3**
⇧ Adults and Larvae Present	⇧ Adults Die	⇧ Unaffected Larvae Mature to Adults	⇧ No Worms Left

Prevention of roundworms involves cleaning up after the puppies often to reduce fecal contamination of the premises. Remember: There are worm eggs shed in the feces, which, after several days, become infective to all dogs. Worming of all the puppies by the breeder, starting as young as two to three weeks, and again three weeks later, will lower the chance of your puppy having worms. Ask your breeder whether your puppy was wormed in this fashion.

Some breeders have a chance to worm their litter only once before selling the puppies. In this case, your vet will have to complete the worming. Have your veterinarian run fecal exams at each visit until the puppy is sixteen weeks old, as not all worms show up on the first or even second fecal exam. Unfortunately, roundworm eggs are not easy to kill once they get into the ground. Normal disinfectant chemicals do not kill them. Direct sunlight and lime will help. Some breeders rotate kennels and runs, which are used for whelping bitches and their litter, to allow time and sunlight to work without any dogs being exposed. Concrete slab flooring is easy to sanitize and make a good surface for limiting roundworms. But this is impractical for the average house pet, and some breeders find it too abrasive for a dog's pads.

> **Public health hazard.** Roundworms can infect people, especially children. The mode of transmission is fecal-oral. This means that the person or child would have to put infected dog feces or fecal-contaminated soil into his or her mouth. The thought is horrifying. But the fact is that young children do these things. Or adults sometimes forget to wash their hands after cleaning up after the puppy. The problem in people is that once the larvae hatch from the eggs in the stomach and small intestine, they get lost trying to find their way. Remember, these larvae are expecting to be in a dog. The lost larvae wind up in the strangest places, like the liver, kidney, brain and eye. Just from their presence, damage to these sites is common. This condition of ascarid larvae in people is called *Toxocariasis*, or *Visceral Larva Migrans*. This should be a serious consideration to all families with young children who have a puppy with roundworms. Consult your physician if this pertains to your situation.

Hookworms

This is another type of intestinal worm parasite of dogs. The worm that infects dogs is called *Ancylostoma caninum*. This worm got its name from the three hook-like teeth it uses to anchor itself to the gut lining. These worms don't just rob their host of food and nutrition like the roundworms; they suck blood—a lot of it. Puppies with a heavy infestation can die from anemia (loss of red blood cells). These worms are very small, measuring only millimeters in length, unlike the roundworms. They are very prolific and congregate in large numbers.

The life cycle of the hookworm is very similar to that of the roundworm. Adult hookworms in the small intestine lay eggs in the gut. These pass out into the environment through the feces. The feces can infect puppies orally, or larvae can hatch from the eggs and burrow through the skin of a puppy. If the egg was ingested, the larvae develop in the intestine. If the larva entered through the skin, it migrates into the bloodstream and ends up in the lungs. From there, it goes into the trachea, gets coughed up and swallowed, and then matures in and infects the intestines.

The four common ways a puppy can become infected with hookworms are these:

1. The puppy eats feces infected with hookworm eggs.

2. A dam bitch can infect her fetuses in utero (in the uterus) if she's infected herself.

3. The dam sheds hookworm larvae in her milk. The puppies become infected during nursing.

4. Third-stage larvae can actually burrow through the tender skin of young puppies, infecting them through this dermal route.

What many breeders find frustrating is that adult dogs can harbor these larvae in their tissues for years. They can be very difficult to exterminate because these larvae are mostly resistant to the drugs we use to worm dogs. Therefore, litter after litter, a bitch can whelp puppies with hookworms even though the bitch was wormed several times with the standard worming drugs. Another factor that propagates the worm burden is the fact that bitches usually lick up the puppy's feces (a cleaning instinct) in a whelping crate. Since most of the puppies are born with worms or get them shortly afterwards through the milk, the dam is reinfecting herself.

Symptoms of a hookworm burden are: anemia with pale mucous membranes; abdominal bloating; excess gas production; foul-smelling, loose diarrhea; bloody stools; emaciated puppies; a poor, dry coat; a chronic cough; an insatiable appetite; and a chronic poor-doer.

The diagnosis of hookworms is made by either of two means: pronounced anemia is seen in a young puppy, without other causes; or the veterinarian performs a fecal exam (called a fecal flotation exam) that visualizes hook-worm eggs under microscopic inspection.

Control of Hookworms. The most common wormers used to kill hook-worms and roundworms are piperazine and pyrantel pamoate. These drugs are given orally. *They kill only the mature adult worms,* so two wormings are needed three weeks apart (that's how long it takes larvae to become adults) to rid a puppy of a worm burden as described in the following chart:

First Worming			Second Worming
⬇			⬇
week 1	**week 2**		**week 3**
⬆	⬆	⬆	⬆
Adults and Larvae Present	Adults Die	Unaffected Larvae Mature to Adults	No Worms Left

Prevention of hookworms involves cleaning up after the puppies often to reduce fecal contamination of the premises. Remember: Worm eggs are shed in the feces, which, after several days, become infective to all dogs. Also, the hookworm larvae can burrow into tender puppy skin if the puppy is allowed to walk through infected feces or contaminated soil. Worming of all the puppies by the breeder, starting as young as two to three weeks and again three weeks later, will lower the chance of your puppy having worms. Ask your breeder whether your puppy was wormed in this fashion.

Some breeders have a chance to worm their litter only once before sell-ing the puppies. In this case, your vet will have to complete the wormings. Have your veterinarian run fecal exams at each visit until the puppy is six-teen weeks old, as not all worms show up on the first or even second fecal exam. Unfortunately, hookworm eggs are not easy to kill once they get into the ground. Normal disinfectant chemicals do not kill them. The larvae are killed by bleach. Direct sunlight and lime can help. Some breeders rotate kennels and runs, which are used for whelping bitches and their litters, to allow time and sunlight to work without any dogs being exposed. Gravel and concrete slab flooring are easy to sanitize and make a good surface for limit-ing hookworms. This is impractical for the average house pet, however, and some breeders find it too abrasive for a dog's pads.

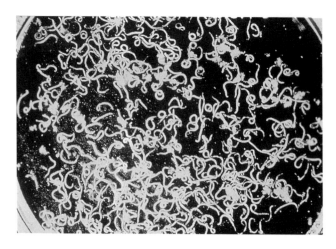

Hookworms.

Public Health Hazard. Like roundworms, hookworms pose a threat to people, especially children. As mentioned earlier, the larvae of the hookworm can burrow through tender foot skin. As children run barefoot in a yard that is contaminated with hookworm larvae, they run the risk of getting hookworm larvae in their skin. This condition is called *Cutaneous Larva Migrans*. These larvae are easily confused, and they become lost trying to find their normal migration route through the lungs. In children, the larvae migrate through the skin. The larvae cause red, raised serpentine eruptions of the skin that are intensely itchy. You can actually see the worms under the skin! Luckily for us, the skin is a dead end for these larvae, but they can cause an allergic reaction. Cats are more often implicated in these cases than dogs. The classic scenario is the family cat using the kids' sandbox as a large litterbox. If the feces of the cat are contaminated with hookworm eggs, the children are at risk.

Whipworms

This small worm lives in the large intestines of dogs. It is shaped like a whip or riding crop. It is only about five centimeters long and very thin. The scientific name for whipworms is *Trichuris vulpis*. These worms attach themselves to the inner lining of the colon, where they feed. Most of the symptoms are from the inflammation of the colon.

The life cycle of the whipworm is very simple and direct compared to those of roundworms and hookworms. Adult whipworms lay eggs while attached in the colon. Larvae develop within the eggs and hatch in two

First Worming		Second Worming	
⇩		⇩	
month 1	**month 2**		**month 3**
⇧	⇧	⇧	⇧
Adults and Larvae Present	Adults Die	Unaffected Larvae Mature to Adults	No Worms Left

weeks. These larvae attach to the inner lining and take another week to develop into adults. Within two to three months, they start laying eggs.

The only way a puppy can become infected is if it eats whipworm eggs in contaminated feces. You may think this is unlikely, but remember that puppies will eat anything. Also, a dog often walks through contaminated feces, then cleans its paws (by licking) and becomes infected. No infection occurs during pregnancy or nursing, as we see with roundworms and hookworms.

The symptoms for whipworms all stem from the colitis (inflammation of the colon) caused by the feeding adult worms. The most common ones are: abdominal bloating and cramping; excess gas; foul-smelling, loose diarrhea; bloody or mucous-coated stools; emaciated puppies; a poor, dry coat; an insatiable appetite; and a chronic poor-doer.

Diagnosis is made by a veterinary examination of a fecal sample, called a fecal flotation exam, which visualizes whipworm eggs under a microscope. The eggs are football-shaped and very distinctive. One or even two negative fecal results doesn't rule out the possibility of whipworms. They are elusive and only show up in fecal exams 30 to 50 percent of the time. If whipworms are suspected, multiple fecal exams should be performed before they are ruled out.

Control of Whipworms. Whipworms are treated by administering anthelmintic drugs (wormers). The most popular drug used now is a powder called Fenbendazole. The powder is mixed in the puppy's food and given for three consecutive days. Due to the two-to-three-month life cycle of the whipworm, a new crop of larvae hatch during that interval. Since there is some question as to whether the larvae are killed along with the adults, many veterinarians repeat the worming in that interval.

The eggs of whipworms are very resistant to chemicals once the eggs get into the environment. Direct sunlight seems to inactivate them. Dogs should be removed from infected areas after being treated for worms. Cleaning up feces daily also helps reduce repeated exposure.

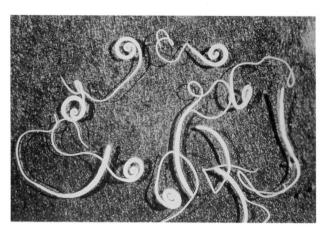

Adult Whipworms. *Dr. D. Bowman*

> **Public Health Hazard.** There doesn't appear to be any public health significance in whipworm infections. People and cats don't get whipworms.

Tapeworms

These internal worms are perhaps the most notorious of all, probably due to the fact that they are the most visible. These flat, white, ribbon-like worms live in the small intestines of many animals, including dogs. They are not in the nematode family of worms like the roundworm or hookworm; they are in a separate group called *Cestodes*. Adult tapeworms are segmented into small sections, each measuring anywhere from to $1/2$ to $1^1/2$ centimeters in length. Most people describe the segments as looking like "grains of white rice" that move! The entire length of an adult worm can be several feet long, as there are hundreds of segments attached in a row. Two different tapeworms infect dogs: *Dipylidium caninum* and *Taenia*. The head of the adult tapeworm is a club-shaped anchor with hooks that attaches to the inner lining of the small intestine.

Tapeworms have an unusual life cycle in that an intermediate host (another creature) is always involved. In the case of *Dipylidium caninum*, it is the common dog and cat flea. In the case of *Taenia*, the intermediate hosts are rodents and rabbits.

Here is a description of the tapeworm life cycle. The head of the adult tapeworm makes segments, each of which is an independent functioning unit that contains packets of eggs. Each segment breaks off one by one and wiggles its way out the host's anus or comes out in the stool. The segments break and release eggs, which fleas, rodents and rabbits may feed on. Once inside the intermediate host, the eggs hatch and a larval tapeworm (called a *cysticercoid*) invades the tissues of the insect or animal. The dog becomes infected by eating a contaminated rodent or rabbit (in the case of *Taenia*) or by swallowing a contaminated flea, as often happens during grooming (in the case of *Dipylidium caninum*). The larva invades the small intestine of the dog, where it develops into an adult.

As mentioned before, a dog can become infected with tapeworms in only two ways:

1. By eating the infected, raw meat of a rodent or rabbit

2. By swallowing an infected flea while grooming itself

The symptoms of tapeworm infection are as follows:

- Weight loss in spite of a voracious appetite
- Rectal itching
- Small, white, rice-grain-like segments in the stool or around the rectum
- Occasional mild abdominal and digestive upsets

Diagnosis is made by observing the tapeworm segments in the dog's stool or stuck to the hairs around the rectum, or by the veterinarian performing an exam on a fecal sample. The eggs are much smaller than those of roundworms, hookworms or whipworms and are very difficult to find. The presence of eggs is a finding inconsistent with tapeworms; therefore, the vast majority of cases are diagnosed by the owner finding the segments on the pet, in its stool or on its bedding. It is important to differentiate between rectal itching from tapeworms and other causes, such as allergic dermatitis and anal gland impaction.

Control of Tapeworms. The key to controlling tapeworms is to eliminate the intermediate host from the picture. In the case of *Taenia* tapeworms, the dog must be kept from eating the raw meat of small wild animals. In the case of *Dipylidium caninum*, you must rid the dog of its flea infestation. This is guaranteed to work, but you may need to continue treatment for one month after ridding the dog of fleas. Treating dogs with tapeworms is easily done with one dose of the drugs Epsiprantel or Praziquantel.

Public Health Hazard. There is very little public health significance for the common dog tapeworms. There have been a few reported cases

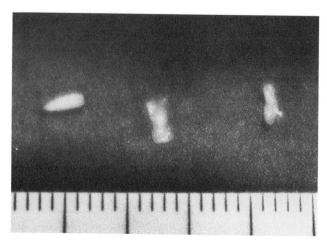

Tapeworm segments .

in children who have eaten fleas off their pet (you can't imagine!). Luckily, this caused no disease or pathology.

We should take a moment to note that a dangerous form of tapeworm exists that can cause serious pathology in people. The tapeworm responsible is *Echinococcus*. Its larvae can cause large tumor-like cysts in the livers, lungs and brains of people. These cysts are called *hydatid cysts*. The tapeworm's intermediate host is sheep. Therefore, people who have sheep should be very careful not to let their dogs eat any raw lamb meat, nor should they consume it themselves.

Heartworm Disease

This is perhaps the most bizarre of the internal parasites of dogs. In heartworm, the parasite is a worm, but instead of it living in the intestines like the other worms described so far, this one lives in the chambers of the heart and in the blood vessels of the lungs. In actuality, then, heartworm is a cardiovascular parasite. Heartworm is found in almost every state in the US, most notably the east coast and southern states. The parasite that causes heartworm is *Dirofilaria immitis*. This worm is spread through the bite of mosquitoes.

The life cycle of heartworm involves an intermediate host—namely, the mosquito. As with all worms, there are adult and larval forms, each one following its own path.

The life cycle of the heartworm begins with the common mosquito biting a dog that has heartworm disease, thus feeding on blood from the dog and becoming infected with the young larvae circulating in the bloodstream, called *microfilariae*. These microfilariae enter the mosquito's digestive tract, molt twice and migrate to the salivary glands as third-stage larvae. When the mosquito bites another dog, it injects these third-stage larvae into the subcutaneous tissues. From there, the larvae molt into fourth-stage larvae and stay in the tissues for about four to five months. The final molt produces the fifth-stage larvae, which migrate into the right side of the heart and pulmonary arteries, where after another month they mature into adults. The adults begin producing microfilariae in two to three months.

You can see it takes about six months from the time a dog is infected with the third-stage larvae for the adults to mature. Only when the adults are present can they reproduce and make microfilariae. The adult worms can get up to several inches in length and look very much like spaghetti. As you can see from the life cycle, the dogs that spend more time outdoors, near wetlands where mosquitoes breed, are far more likely to contract heartworm disease. *Dogs become infected with heartworm disease through the bite of an infected common mosquito.*

From twenty-five to one hundred of the adult worms can live in the heart and lungs of a dog at any one time. You can imagine how they would clog up the heart valves and blood vessels to the lungs. Most of the symptoms of heartworm disease stem from this phenomenon. Please note that symptoms don't usually begin for several months to three years after infection, as it takes this long for the adults to occupy the heart and start causing congestive heart failure and obstructive pulmonary disease.

The common symptoms are a chronic, persistent cough; general body weakness; loss of weight; exercise intolerance; fluid accumulation in the liver and abdomen; dilated pulmonary blood vessels; venous dilation and congestion; and kidney disease due to damage of the glomerulus filtering system.

The diagnosis of heartworm disease can be accomplished in several different ways. Each enables a veterinarian to identify either the microfilariae that circulate in the bloodstream or the adults that live in the right side of the heart (mostly the right atrium) and in the blood vessels of the lungs. Of the four different tests available, we recommend the Occult Antigen test. It is by far the most accurate. A sample of venous blood is taken, allowed to clot, and spun down in a centrifuge to separate the blood cells from the serum. The serum is then tested using an ELISA (Enzyme-Linked Immunosorbent Assay), which tests for the most minute levels of microfilariae or adult worm antigen (proteins on the surface of the parasite). This means of testing for heartworm is the most popular now because we realize that up to 15 percent of heartworm infections never produce the microfilariae. We call these cases occult (hidden). Therefore, if you are using a test that only tests for their presence, the test is intrinsically only 85 percent accurate. The ELISA tests approach 98 percent accuracy. The cost is more, but you can't argue with the value.

If a dog is symptomatic with a persistent cough, a chest X ray will reveal a distended right atrium of the heart and pulmonary blood vessels. An electrocardiogram will also demonstrate an enlarged right atrium. A physical exam can reveal a heart murmur.

Control of Heartworm Disease

This disease is much easier to prevent than it is to treat. If a dog is mainly indoors, exposure to mosquitoes will be limited. Even when windows have screens, however, these little obstinate flying hypodermic needles still get into the home. Therefore, it is our recommendation that all puppies receive a heartworm prevention medication when as young as eight weeks of age. Two different types of heartworm prevention medications are available: one that needs to be given daily and one that is given monthly. Many different brands are on the market, but all of them fit into one of these two categories:

Daily Prevention. These medications must be given daily. They kill only the third-stage infective larvae. Since the third-stage larvae can molt into fourth-stage larvae within one day, the medication must be given daily to work. The main ingredient is diethylcarbamazine. This is effective and safe for use in puppies. These medications are inexpensive and have been used widely for decades. They come in various forms, including tablets, chewable wafers and syrup. However, if a dog with heartworm disease and circulating microfilariae is given diethylcarbamazine, many of the microfilariae will die, causing a sudden antigen overload. This can precipitate a fatal shock. All dogs must be tested negative for heartworm prior to being given any type of heartworm prevention.

Monthly Prevention. These medications kill the third- through fifth-stage tissue larvae, so they can be given once a month. The different stages of larvae are killed before they can mature into adults, thus preventing heartworm disease. Each medication contains a different active ingredient. The first medication contains Ivermectin and comes in three sizes: for small dogs (one to twenty-five pounds), for medium dogs (twenty-six to fifty pounds), and for large dogs (fifty-one to 100 pounds). Giant dogs over 100 pounds need a combination of sizes. Originally, a precautionary statement in the package insert warned users about Ivermectin overdoses in Collies, with the possibility of neurological side effects and toxicity, including ataxia, drooling, coma and

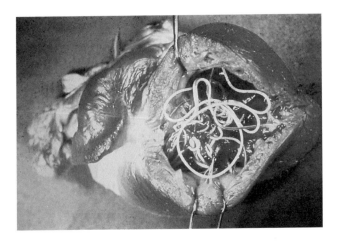

Adult Heartworms in heart chamber. *Dr. D. Bowman*

death. Currently, manufacturers claim a wide margin of safety in Collies when the recommended dosage level is not exceeded.

The other monthly heartworm preventive on the market has the active ingredient milbemycin oxime. It works by killing the tissue larval stages of the heartworm. This ingredient also has been shown to kill other internal parasites, such as adult roundworms, hookworms and whipworms. It comes in four sizes: for toy dogs (one to ten pounds), for small dogs (eleven to twenty-five pounds), for medium dogs (twenty-six to fifty pounds), and for large dogs (fifty-one to 100 pounds). Giant dogs (those over 100 pounds) need a combination of sizes.

Because both monthly preventatives can kill the microfilariae that circulate in the bloodstream, you must use the occult heartworm antigen test, which doesn't depend on finding these microfilariae but tests for the presence of the parasite.

Many people like the daily medication because it's cheaper and has been used for many years, while others prefer the monthly medication because of its convenience and broad spectrum features. Regardless of the type of prevention used, there are a few guidelines to remember:

- It is preferable to keep your puppy on heartworm prevention all year round, especially if you live in a warm climate where mosquitoes are out continually. Many people in colder climates are starting to do this also.
- If your puppy is on heartworm prevention all year round, he should still have an annual heartworm test. Studies have shown that up to 14 percent of the dogs that supposedly received their preventive pill

didn't actually get it for one reason or another (it wasn't swallowed, or it was vomited up).

- If you live in a climate that has winters which eliminate the mosquitoes, you can stop the preventive two months after the first hard frost and start back up again one month before the first mosquito appears. But remember that you must test for heartworm before starting up again.

- If you skip more than a week of daily heartworm prevention or more than thirty days of the monthly heartworm prevention, your puppy should be tested prior to your starting up again.

- Because all heartworm preventives are dosed according to the weight of your puppy, if you have a breed that is quickly growing and changing its weight every week, it may be wise to start the puppy on a chewable daily prevention, which is easy to dose until his weight stabilizes, then switch over to a monthly one. This switchover must be done within thirty days from stopping the daily prevention.

In the unfortunate event of your puppy contracting heartworm disease, an early diagnosis is crucial to a favorable outcome. This is one reason an annual heartworm test is recommended (if you don't use preventive on your puppy, it is crucial to have him tested twice a year). Once the diagnosis is made, your veterinarian will discuss treatment options. The drug most often used to kill the adult worms is an arsenic-based compound (yes, arsenic!) called sodium thiacetarsamide. This drug must be given slowly by intravenous injection over a two-day period. This is like a form of chemotherapy because the dog can become quite ill during the process, which is why most vets do blood tests prior to starting treatment so that they can check the general health status of the patient. Other routine pre-treatment tests are chest X rays, an electrocardiogram and, sometimes, an echocardiogram. All the information obtained by these diagnostic tests helps the veterinarian assess the condition of the patient and ensures a more accurate prognosis.

Immediately following the intravenous drug therapy, the puppy must have absolute rest. Remember that dozens of dead worms are breaking up and floating around in the heart and pulmonary arteries. It is very easy for these to break off and cause an embolism in the lungs. Therefore, the puppy must be kept very quiet for several weeks after the treatment. Most veterinarians order cage rest and use buffered aspirin as an anti-embolism drug during this stage.

Several weeks after the treatment for the adult worms, medication must be given to kill the circulating microfilariae in the blood. Different medications are available for this purpose. The older drug is dithiazanine iodide, which is given for a week. More recently, the monthly heartworm preventives are being used to kill the microfilariae. We have used both with good results.

If the puppy is strong and healthy without other complicating diseases or conditions, and if the disease is diagnosed early (within a year), treatment is more likely to succeed. In these cases, the prognosis is *fair* to *good*. Poor health, congenital heart defects, malnutrition, concomitant disease, old age or a delay in making the diagnosis will all worsen the prognosis.

Coccidia

This parasite belongs to an entirely different group of parasites than the worms described in the preceding sections. These are *protozoan*, the same group of microscopic creatures amoebas belong to. Coccidia are parasitic one-celled microscopic organisms and they are also *species specific*. The genus of coccidia that infects dogs is *Isospora*.

The life cycle of coccidia is relatively complex, involving several forms of the organism. The coccidia eggs (called *oocysts*) pass out in the feces of infected animals.

It is clear from the description of this life cycle that dogs become infected with coccidia by oral contamination with feces from infected animals.

All this invasion and destruction of intestinal epithelial cells causes an inflammation of the intestinal lining, called *enteritis*. The puppies most susceptible to coccidia are those under stress (involving shipping, overcrowding, pet shops, etc.). The symptoms of coccidia are loose or watery stools; bloody stools; vomiting; malnutrition; abdominal bloating; weight loss; and straining to defecate.

Not all animals with coccidia are symptomatic; they are called *carriers*. If the dam bitch is a carrier, all the puppies in her litter will be exposed. The weakest of the puppies will come down with the worst cases.

> **Control of Coccidia.** Control of this disease stems from the identification of all carrier animals in a kennel or household. All infected feces must be cleaned up. All infected dogs must be treated. Treatment is very easy and effective with sulfonamide antibiotics.

Giardia

Giardia canis is another protozoan that infects dogs. These one-celled organisms are free-living in outdoor water sources, such as ponds, streams and brooks. What's different about these protozoa is that they have a whip-like tail that propels them, called a *flagella*. Many different protozoa have this tail, and they are collectively called *flagellates*. When these giardia are free-living outdoors, they cause no harm. But when a dog becomes infected, they cause intestinal disease.

The life cycle of giardia is very simple. There are only two forms, or stages. The infective stage of the giardia is called a *cyst*; it is like an egg. Once swallowed by a dog (from an outdoor water source, for example), the infective cyst "hatches" and releases the adult form, called a *trophozoite*. It is this form that has the flagella tail. These are mobile and make their way to the small intestine. There they colonize the mucosal lining of the intestine, causing inflammation. They populate and release more cysts that pass out in the feces.

Dogs become infected with giardia by ingesting outdoor water or feces of animals that contain the infective cyst.

The various and sometimes nebulous symptoms of giardia infections are chronic and persistent diarrhea; loose and mucous-coated stools; abdominal bloating; weight loss; and chronic poor-doer.

The diagnosis of giardia occurs through the identification of the parasite from the sick puppy. This can be accomplished in one of three ways:

1. The veterinarian performs a fecal flotation fecal exam under a high-power microscope to visualize the giardia cysts.

2. The veterinarian may perform a rectal swab, which takes some fresh feces and rectal mucus directly from the rectum, and immediately examines it for the presence of the trophozoite form. This procedure is called a *direct smear*.

3. A new test is available that can detect a very small amount of the parasite in feces. It is an ELISA test and is very sensitive and very specific for giardia.

Control of Giardia. The best way to control giardia is to limit exposure to outside water sources. This is clearly difficult if your dog swims or is used for sport. During these sessions, bring clean drinking water so that your puppy can drink that when it gets thirsty. The other way to avoid contracting this disease is to keep your puppy from eating wild animal droppings. This make sense when you consider that all wild animals drink outdoor water. Most wild mammals have giardia in their bowels. They also pass the infective cysts out in their droppings. These animals are generally resistant to the protozoan. Deer droppings appear to be a common reservoir. When your dog comes across a nice fresh pile of deer droppings, keep it from devouring them!

The treatment of giardia in dogs involves anti-protozoal drugs. One of the most popular of these is metronidazole. These drugs should be used for a short time only (about five days), or side effects can be noted, the most common being neurological symptoms and inner ear disturbances. These manifest as dizziness and loss of balance. As mentioned, this parasite is very difficult to diagnose, so most vets treat for it if there is a presumptive diagnosis of giardia with chronic mucous diarrhea.

Public Health Hazard. People can become infected if they drink outside water without boiling it first. (We will assume that nobody consumes wild or domestic animal feces.) People with young children should not allow them to crawl through the puppy's feces for many reasons, the least of which is the possibility of contracting giardia.

Chapter 4

Preventive Health Maintenance

This chapter deals with the basics of preventive health and daily maintenance of your puppy, from cleaning and grooming to feeding and basic nutrition. We will also briefly touch on topics like some home remedies, holistic alternatives, spaying and neutering and pet health insurance.

This mixed bag of information is a collection of veterinary tidbits, along with generally accepted puppy-rearing practices. It's an accumulation of advice from breeders, dog handlers, groomers, animal health technicians, veterinarians and dog enthusiasts. The chapter is divided into five sections:

1. Maintenance of Specific Body Parts (teeth and gums, ears, eyes, nails, coat)
2. Feeding and Nutrition
3. Spaying and Neutering
4. Home Remedies and Holistic Alternatives
5. Pet Health Insurance

Maintenance of Specific Body Parts
Tooth and Gum Care

Teeth are just as important to your puppy as they are to you—maybe more so. After all, we don't use our teeth to hold, carry and play with our toys. We don't generally use them to protect ourselves either. We use our teeth to chew food (and maybe fingernails, if you're the nervous type). I guess smiling counts, too.

If we lose our teeth, we have the option of getting dentures, which don't really affect our lives too much, except that we have to be more careful about what we eat. But if a dog loses its teeth, not only is eating difficult, but there go the tug-of-war games, retrieving, chewing bones or furniture and self-defense. Just about everything a dog lives for!

I think you get the point: A dog's dentition is definitely worth protecting and saving. New veterinary dental procedures can include endodontics and bonding. Before we learn how to keep our dog's teeth healthy, let's first look into things we humans do to protect our teeth. On a daily basis, most of us do at least one, if not a combination of, the following: brush, use mouthwash, floss, use water picks, get professional cleaning and get regular dental checkups.

What is the point? We just wanted to illustrate some of the different ways we humans try to hold onto our teeth as long as possible. Now, just imagine if you did *nothing*. How long do you think your teeth would last? Well, history tells us there were days gone by when people didn't really do anything preventive to keep their teeth; consequently, they *expected* to lose them in their early adulthood. Their teeth just rotted away.

Obviously, animals don't do anything to clean their teeth. They go through their entire lives without doing as much as brushing, ever. Consequently, many dogs begin losing their teeth in mid-life. One by one, usually starting with the front incisors, they fall out. Just take a look at a seven-year-old dog's teeth. Unless he's unusual, there will be lots of tartar, discoloration, odor, black areas of decay (a cavity or caries) and probably cracked or missing teeth.

Now, let's be fair about this. Animals in general have a higher resistance to tooth decay for several reasons. First, their saliva is more resistant to bacterial growth than ours is. Saliva is one of the main natural defenses against tooth decay. It keeps the pH in the mouth high (an alkaline environment), which decreases tooth enamel erosion from bacterial growth and the acid the bacteria produce. A tooth starts to decay only when a hole is eroded through the enamel or if bacteria travels between the gum and tooth root and decays or abscesses the root itself. Second, dogs generally chew on harder things than we do. This mechanical scraping helps keep tartar from accumulating. Third, the enamel coating of a dog's teeth is generally thicker than ours.

Despite these positive things going for them, without basic dental care, dogs will end up with tooth decay, tooth rot, cavities, root abscesses, cracked teeth, periodontal disease and, ultimately, tooth loss.

Before we go on, it is time to define some dental terminology so that you understand the basic processes of dental disease. Many of you will recognize some of these terms, as many pertain to people as well.

Glossary of Dental Terms

Alveolar bone. This is the bone of the skull (for upper teeth) or jaw (for lower teeth) in which the roots of the teeth sit.

Caries. The erosion and destruction of tooth enamel and dentine, which produces a crater in the tooth. This is usually done by acid produced by bacteria in plaque and tartar. Also known as a cavity.

Cementum. This is the connective tissue that anchors the tooth root to its socket in the alveolar bone.

Crown. The part of the tooth that is above the gum line (the part you can see). Most of the crown is covered by enamel.

Dentine. The majority of the bulk of a tooth. It is found just below the enamel and is also hard, but not nearly as much as the enamel. If the enamel cracks or erodes, the dentine will be exposed to the air.

Enamel. The white or off-white hard substance that covers and protects the deeper structures of a tooth. This is what gives a tooth its white color and high gloss. It is the hardest substance in the body.

Periodontal disease. Also known as *periodontitis.* This is an inflammation of the tissues around and that support the teeth, such as the gums, alveolar bone and connective tissue. This usually starts from an accumulation of plaque and tartar between the crown of the tooth and surrounding tissues, causing a separation of the tooth and its socket, and allowing bacteria and infection to further detach the tooth from its socket. This process eventually leads to tooth loss.

Periodontal ligament. More connective tissue that anchors the tooth root to its socket.

Plaque. A sticky film comprised of bacteria, saliva, white blood cells and mineral deposits.

Pulp cavity. This is the sensitive center to a tooth that contains the dental nerve, artery and vein. This fleshy center has feeling and bleeds if disrupted.

Tartar (dental calculus). A hard yellow to grayish-green mineralized coating on teeth comprised of saliva, plaque, minerals, food particles and bacteria. Tartar is one of the main causes of periodontal disease.

Tooth abscess. A pocket of infection around the roots of a tooth and the alveolar socket, causing pain, swelling, bleeding, pus formation and, eventually, tooth loss.

Tooth roots. These are the finger-like projections at the base of a tooth that carry the dental nerve and blood vessels to the pulp cavity, and are seated into the alveolar bone.

Here's a flowchart of what can happen if you totally ignore your puppy's teeth: Eating primarily canned, wet or human food encourages plaque formation. If not removed, plaque mineralizes into tartar within a week. Slowly, over months and years, the tartar causes a recession of the gum line and separation of the tooth root from its socket in the alveolar bone. If left untreated, this separation continues until the root of the tooth is exposed and loose. At this point, there is usually much green tartar accumulated and horrible halitosis (bad breath), and tooth loss is almost inevitable.

What a horrible scenario! There must be a way of preventing this from happening. What are the steps one can take to prevent such a tragedy, you ask? We thought you'd never ask. Here are the main steps you can take now, while your puppy is young, to help ensure many years of a beautiful healthy smile:

First, **look at your puppy's teeth**. See how clean, white and glossy they are? The gums are healthy, with no evidence of disease. That's the way they should look for the life of your dog; like pearls!

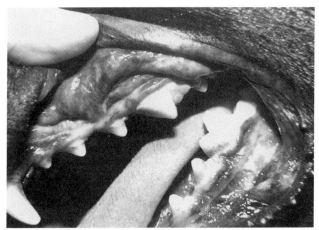

Tartar appears as a yellow to grayish-green coating on the teeth.

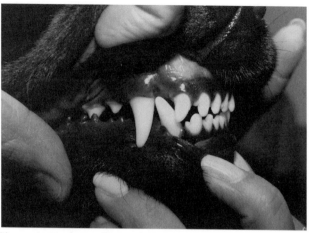

Normal, healthy teeth. See how white and glossy they are and how healthy the gums look?

Dry is better. Feed your puppy a high-quality, dry kibble food. Only use canned food or table scraps as treats. The kibble will help keep teeth clean.

Brush your puppy's teeth at least twice weekly. This can be done easily with one of your old toothbrushes and baking soda. Add just enough water to two tablespoons of baking soda to make it pasty. Spread the paste onto the head of the toothbrush or directly onto the outer surfaces of the teeth. You'll have to lift up the lips to do this. You also can use commercially available doggie toothpaste and toothbrushes. *If your puppy is introduced to this procedure early on, it won't be a struggle later in life.* The key is to start at the gum line and brush downward in a circular motion. Concentrate on the outer surfaces, as this is where most of the tartar and plaque accumulate. Brush vigorously for two minutes. If your puppy gets tired sooner, take a short rest, then continue. No rinsing is needed. You can get away with brushing only once or twice a week because, unlike human plaque, puppy plaque takes several days to mineralize into tartar. Dentists tell us that our plaque needs only twenty-four hours to do that, hence the "at least once a day" rule. Obviously, the more you brush, the healthier the teeth and gums will be.

Finger toothbrushes are available. If you want to "brush" your dog's teeth with your finger, you can buy small, rubberized, knobby finger toothbrushes, or you can wrap a piece of gauze over your finger and use that.

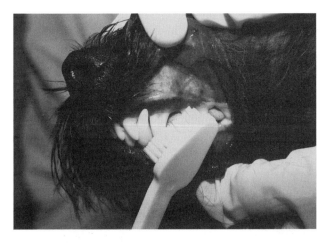

Brush your puppy's teeth at least twice a week. The more you brush, the healthier the teeth and gums will be.

Hygiene spray. Think of hygiene sprays as mouthwash for dogs. These are formulated to be sprayed or swabbed onto your dog's teeth daily. They help kill bacteria and neutralize odors, and some contain fluoride. These don't need rinsing.

Enzyme-coated rawhides. Most puppies like to chew. Hopefully, they chew on the right things. You can take advantage of that behavior and let them chew on something that helps clean their teeth. You can buy strips of beef hide impregnated with an enzyme that retards bacterial growth. Giving one of these a few times a week may decrease plaque formation. My dog loves them.

Professional Cleaning. This is done by a veterinarian and his or her staff, and involves a combination of hand scaling as well as an ultrasonic unit to literally blast tartar off. The process is a bit tedious, and it must be done slowly. All surfaces must be scaled to remove even the smallest amount of tartar from all surfaces of the tooth. Each tooth is scaled separately. Once all teeth are done, they need to be polished with a tooth polish. The reason is that during the scaling, microscopic lines are made in the enamel. If these aren't smoothed out by polishing, then they will provide places for tartar to accumulate. Scaling is recommended when you notice tartar buildup, or yearly as part of a prevention program.

Many veterinarians require that your puppy be anesthetized with a general anesthetic during the scaling. This enables them to get around

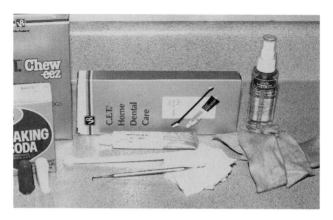

This assortment of teeth-cleaning products for dogs includes treats, baking soda, finger toothbrushes, a regular toothbrush, "doggie" toothpaste, a dental pick, oral hygiene spray, and enzyme-coated rawhides.

each tooth and do a more thorough job. This is fine; however, it is possible to use a mild sedative instead. Although this may seem awkward for the vet, and it certainly takes more time and patience, the puppy isn't subjected to general anesthesia. *The less anesthesia given to a young puppy, the better, especially if it's done on a regular basis.*

Following at least two or three of the preceding steps will greatly increase your puppy's chances of keeping the beautiful set of teeth it was born with its whole life. My dog is now eleven years old, and, boy, what a smile he has, just like on the day I got him!

Ear Care

Ears come in all different shapes and sizes in dogs. Compare the cropped, erect ears of a Doberman Pinscher with the long, floppy ears of a Basset Hound. Each ear is different; a puppy can have a left ear that's always having problems, while the right one is fine. Even dogs within a breed can be different. For example, I've seen certain Miniature Schnauzers that constantly get ear infections, and others that never have a problem. Go figure. The point is that each dog and each ear is different, and you shouldn't generalize. But one of my jobs in this book is to make recommendations that pertain to the average case.

To begin with, let's review the basic anatomy of an ear. On the outside is the ear flap, or *pinna*. This is a flap of cartilage sandwiched between two layers of skin. All ears are assembled the same regardless of the size, shape or breed. At the junction of the pinna and the skull, the ear turns into a conical tunnel called the *outer ear canal*. It has two parts: the vertical and horizontal canals. Think of the ear canal as an inverted "L." At the bottom of the horizontal canal lies the *tympanic membrane*, or eardrum. This membrane separates the outer ear from the middle ear.

Our discussion will be only of the ear flap and outer ear canal. Problems of the middle and inner ear are addressed in other chapters.

Care of the Ear Flap

Following are descriptions of three of the most common ailments of the ear flap. The first one (cropping) is man-made, as it is a surgical procedure many veterinarians are still performing. The second (bites) is caused by flies that bite and suck blood. The third (frostbite) is also a man-made condition; this is what happens when a dog is left out in subfreezing weather without enough shelter.

Cropped Ears. Very little maintenance actually is needed for a healthy ear flap in breeds where the flap is kept natural. In puppies where the breed dictates cropping, the veterinary surgeon will crop the ear in a standard pattern for the breed at about twelve weeks of age. Antibiotics may be dispensed following surgery, to prevent infection. The skin margins often bleed and ooze serum for several days after surgery. Many breeders then tape the ears if the breed calls for erect ears. Taping means that the cropped ear is kept in an upright, erect posture with use of a cotton support rod taped into the outer ear canal. Then a piece of tape is used between the ears to form a bridge that keeps the ears vertical.

There is some controversy regarding ear cropping. Some breeders and dog enthusiasts believe this procedure is cruel and unnecessary. They also feel the same about tail docking (although it's not quite the same, as tail docking is done at two days of age). In fact, there are European countries that have outlawed the procedures. I don't mean to get into the debate any further, other than to raise the issue.

Fly Bites. Several different flies bite the ear flaps of dogs: black fly, may fly, deer fly and horsefly. These flies love the inside of tender young ear flaps. In many parts of the country, these biting flies come out in the spring—for instance, the may fly comes out in April or May. These fly bites leave large welts that itch and bleed. These bites most often occur on the flap tip. These can be treated with topical antibiotics and cortisone ointments. The prevention is to limit the puppies' outside exposure during the fly months or to apply a fly repellent to the ear flaps before turning the dog out. Anything that attracts flies should be removed, such as fertilizer or compost piles.

Frostbite. One of the most common sites for frostbite in dogs is the tip of the ear flap. The reason is that there is reduced blood flow and less hair there. Dogs left in bitterly cold weather (usually subfreezing) for hours are at risk. Frostbite literally means the freezing and killing of tissue. Initially, the skin turns white and loses feeling. Once the dog is brought inside, the skin starts to thaw, at which time it becomes very red and painful due to the tremendous inflammatory response in the damaged skin. After a few days, the dead skin starts to turns black and dry up. We call this *devitalization* of the tissue. The junction of vital (living) skin and dead skin forms a visible *line of demarcation*.

If frostbite is diagnosed, the veterinarian slowly thaws out the skin with warm water bottles. The skin that is still viable will survive. The skin that died is surgically removed after a waiting period of two to four weeks. The surgeon should take every step to preserve as much of the remaining flap as possible.

Care of the Outer Ear Canal

The first thing we'll do is go through the common causes of outer ear canal problems. By far, the most common problem we see in the ear canal is infection. Most people refer to these as ear infections. We will be more accurate and call them infections of the outer ear canal, or *otitis externa*. There are three basic types of outer ear infections:

1. Ear mite infections

2. Bacterial infections

3. Yeast infections

The environment of the ear canal is very important in encouraging the growth of bacteria or yeast. If the ear canal is dry and clean, and air gets in readily, then bacteria and yeast cannot grow. The environment needed to grow bacteria and yeast is dark, damp and warm, and has a reduced air flow.

Let's take a closer look at otitis externa. Realize that it usually takes a veterinarian to be able to differentiate between the bacterial and yeast etiologies. Their clinical presentation can look very similar. In fact, we often need to do a culture of the ear canal to see what's growing.

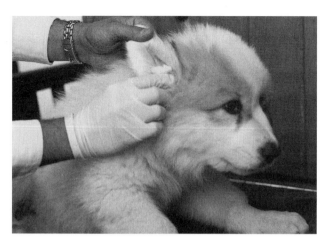

You can clean your puppy's ears at home. Follow the guidelines in this chapter to do them properly. *Arlene Oraby*

Ear Mites. A full description of ear mites is given in Chapter 2.

Bacterial Otitis Externa. Bacterial ear canal infections are very common in puppies, especially those that swim often or get frequent baths. Certain bacteria commonly reside in the ear canal. If the con-ditions are right for the bacteria to multiply, bacterial growth will flourish, resulting in enough to cause disease. We call this an *overgrowth* of bacteria. A veterinarian usually needs to culture the ear canal to get an identification. Also, a sensitivity report should be done. This is part of the culture report, and it lists the appropriate antibiotics that will kill the specific bacteria grown in the culture. (For a complete description of bacterial ear infections, please see Chapter 6, "Puppy Pediatrics.")

Some cases of otitis externa become chronic, or prolonged. The breeds most prone to chronic ear infections are those with long, floppy ear flaps that hang down and cover the opening to the ear canal. Some of these breeds are the spaniels, retrievers, hounds, poodles and any dog that routinely swims. If you have a puppy that already is developing a chronic ear problem, you may want to follow some of the preventive measures described later in this section.

Yeast Otitis Externa. Yeast is the budding form of fungus. A certain amount of yeast normally lives in the ears of dogs. Remember, the environment that encourages yeast growth is dark, damp and warm, with reduced air flow. If water gets trapped in the outer ear canal, the yeast will start to flourish. This happens during swimming and bathing. (For a complete description of yeast ear infections, please see Chapter 6, "Puppy Pediatrics.")

Any dog that swims regularly or is bathed frequently runs a high risk of getting water down the ear canal, which predisposes it to yeast otitis externa.

How to Keep the Ear Healthy

The following is a list of steps you can take to prevent ear disease. Not all of these need to be done concurrently; all you may need is one or two of the steps. Ask your veterinarian which ones pertain to your puppy.

Pluck That Hair. One of the most common causes of outer ear problems is excess hair in the outer ear canal. All dogs have some hair in their ear canals, but certain breeds have more than their share, such as the Miniature Schnauzer, all varieties of Poodles, the Lhasa Apso, the Shih Tzu and the Bichon Frise. What the hair does is keep the ear wax from working its way out of the ear canal. In effect, it traps it like a wick. As was mentioned previously, wax accumulation coupled with warmth, dampness, darkness and a lack of air circulation leads to ear infections. Most groomers pluck out the ear hair as part of grooming, so many breeds have it done every four to six weeks. At home, you can pluck out hairs with your fingertips slowly, a few hairs at a time. As you can imagine, your puppy may not take to this too kindly, but just remember that not all things that are good for you are fun. Groomers and veterinarians often use tweezers or a pointy-nosed hemostat instead of fingers. If the plucking is done properly, your puppy will suffer minimal discomfort. Have your groomer or veterinarian show you how to do it.

Regular Ear Cleanings. Your vet can clean your puppy's ears occasionally, but for cleanings to be of any real benefit, *you* should clean the ears weekly. Use a commercially prepared dog ear cleaner. It should have a ceruminolytic agent to break up the wax. Some have menthol and eucalyptus extracts to soothe the irritated ear canal. A few have antiseptic agents to discourage bacterial and yeast growth. If your puppy has wet ears, use an ear cleaner that has an astringent (drying agent). As you may find out, dozens of ear cleaners are on the market. Ask your vet which one is best for your puppy, or follow this chart:

Which Type of Ear Cleaner to Use					
Type of Problem	Surfactant (soap)	Ceruminolytic (dissolves wax)	Soothing Extracts	Antiseptic Agents	Astringents
Just Plain Dirty	X				
Waxy Ears	X	X			
Sour Odor, no Wax	X			X	
Sour Odor & Wax	X	X		X	
Clean but Red	X		X		
Bacterial Infection	X		X	X	
Yeast Infection	X		X	X	X
Frequent Baths & Swimming					X X

Regardless of which cleaner you use, the technique is the same. I like to use cotton on a roll. Use the guidelines that follow here and onto the next page:

1. Tear off a piece of cotton about two inches long.

2. Soak the cotton in the ear cleaner you have chosen.

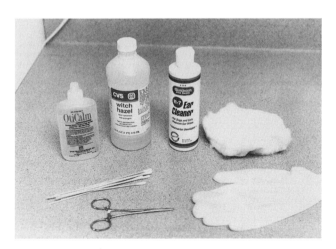

An ear-cleaning kit can include a cleansing solution, witch hazel, cotton, long swabs, hair tweezers and rubber gloves for hygiene.

3. Using your finger, gently swab the inside of the ear canal with the wet cotton.

4. Use circular motions to wipe out the ear canal.

5. If there is a large accumulation of dirt or wax, pour the cleaner into the ear canal, massage it in with your hand, and then swab out the ear canal with dry cotton.

6. *Never use cotton-tipped swabs*, as these can damage the eardrum if improperly angled.

7. Continue until no more dirt comes out with the swabbing. It may take a dozen or more swabbings to clean a dirty ear.

8. Do the same for the other ear.

Keep Those Ears Dry. If your puppy likes to swim or must be bathed frequently, he runs an increased risk of developing ear problems. Place cotton in the outer ear canals to keep water out. If that's impossible, rinse the ear canals with an astringent after swimming or bathing, to dry the ear and remove any residual water.

How to Medicate Ears

The procedure for cleaning ears is described in the previous section. Medicating ears is a little different. In most situations, a thorough cleaning of the ear is necessary prior to applying any medication. After all, placing medication on top of wax or infectious debris doesn't do much good.

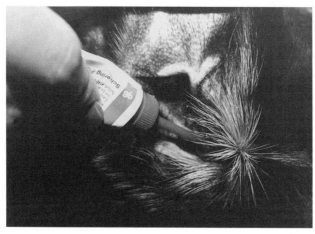

Applying ointment in the puppy's ear.

Most ear medications are in the form of ointments. These are a bit greasy, but they make good vehicles for delivering the active ingredients to the site. Applying ointment into an ear canal is a simple procedure, once you know how. Follow these instructions:

1. Make sure the ointment you're using hasn't expired. You can find the expiration date on the crimp (end) of the tube.

2. Make sure the ears are clean. If they're not, read the preceding section on cleaning the ear.

3. Hold up the ear flap so that the opening to the external ear canal is visible.

4. Most ear ointments have a tip or nozzle. While holding the tube upside-down and vertical, insert the tip into the canal opening only as far as you can see.

5. You should squirt enough ointment into the ear canal to fill it. You will see it welling back up at you. This can be anywhere from five drops in a Yorkshire Terrier to twenty-five drops in a Saint Bernard.

6. Thoroughly massage the ointment into the ear canal so that it works its way down to the bottom. Remember, the ear canal is in the shape of an inverted "L."

Eye Care

The eye is a complicated anatomical structure. For the purposes of this chapter, we will focus on normal maintenance of a healthy eye. Other than traumatic injury to the eye, the majority of eye afflictions are in the form of inflammations and infections of the tissues surrounding the eye.

When we say the "eye," we really mean the three main components of the eye: the *globe* of the eye, the *eyelids* (upper, lower, and nictitans); and the *conjunctiva*, or tissues surrounding the globe.

The *globe* of the eye is the eyeball itself. The upper and lower eyelids are skin with eyelashes projecting from the outer margins. The *nictitans*, or third eyelid, is a protective veil the dog can raise to cover the surface of the eyeball (also called the *cornea*). The third eyelid has a slip of cartilage in it to keep its shape and rigidity, and a gland of the nictitans that acts as a lymph node to fight infection and secrete lubrication. The *conjunctiva* is the mucous membrane that surrounds the eyeball. This is the pink tissue that gets very red and swollen in a case of *pinkeye* and *conjunctivitis*.

Care of the Eyelids, Conjunctiva and Eyeball

The eyelids are basically skin structures. Therefore, the problems of the lids are those of skin. Congenital eye defects such as entropion (an inward rolling of the lower eyelid), ectropion (an outward rolling of the lower eyelid) and cherry eye were described in Chapter 1. This section covers common ailments of the eyelids and the steps you can take to keep them healthy.

The conjunctiva is a mucous membrane of tissue that surrounds the eyeball and fills the space between the eyeball and eyelid. It is pink and wet. When the eye becomes irritated, the conjunctiva swells and becomes red. There may also be a discharge from it. Unlike the clear watery discharge from irritated eyes, the discharge from infected eyes is usually thick and yellow. (For a complete description of the diseases of the eyes, please see Chapter 6, " Puppy Pediatrics.")

How to Keep Those Eyes Bright

The preceding list illustrates how many different things can go wrong with the eyes and how important it is to maintain healthy eyes. Some of these conditions are hard to prevent, such as when an accident happens and trauma to the eye occurs especially if you have a breed with pronounced eyes. But you can keep some of these things from happening. Following is a list:

- Keep hair cut short around the eyes so that it doesn't get into the eyes and irritate them.

- If your puppy is one that has a lot of crusty discharge, wipe it away frequently. Use warm water on a washcloth or tissue. Wipe in a downward motion so that you don't run the risk of poking the eye. You may need to do this daily in some breeds, like the Poodle, Lhasa Apso, Shih Tzu and Pekingese.

- Keep your puppy from lunging face-first into bushes and plants, as they can get poked in the eye by the branches.

- Avoid playing any rough games that could involve trauma to the eye, such as throwing sticks or pointed objects for your puppy to catch. Only use smooth, rounded or soft play things like tennis balls, Frisbees or soft handballs.

- Reduce the irritants in your home and yard that may cause eye irritation. Some of the things that are very irritating to a puppy's eyes are dust, paint and adhesive fumes, sawdust and plaster dust, indoor plants, mold spores, city soot, aerosol spray propellants, carpet

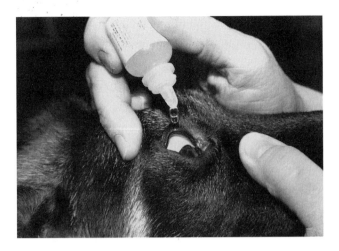

To apply drops, gently pull back the upper eyelid.

cleaners, certain fabric fibers, outdoor pollens and grass cuttings, dried soil and car exhaust.

- Have your puppy checked routinely for internal parasites, as some of them can cause eye damage.

- Avoid physical contact with other dogs or cats that have mange, ringworm or any skin ailment of unknown cause.

- Never hit your dog in the face or head for fear of causing eye trauma (you shouldn't be doing that kind of thing anyway).

- At the first sign of redness, hair loss around the eyes, swelling of the conjunctiva or eyelids, eye itching or any watery or thick discharge of the eyes, consult your veterinarian!

Applying Eye Medication

Two basic types of ophthalmic medications are commonly applied to the eyes: drops and ointment. Following are directions for applying each of these to the eye:

Drops. To apply an eye drop to the eye, raise your puppy's nose upward about 30 degrees. Gently pull back the upper lid so that the white of the eye is showing. Drop one drop onto the white of the eye. Hold the nose up for ten seconds.

Ointment. To apply ointment to the eye, raise your puppy's nose upward about 30 degrees. Gently pull down the lower lid so that a pocket

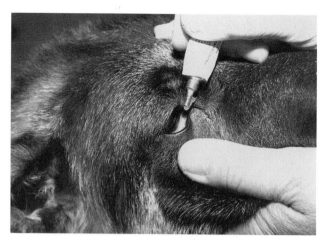

To apply ointment, gently pull down the lower lid.

forms between the lower lid and the conjunctiva. Squeeze one-quarter inch of ointment into the pocket. Let go of the lower lid, and allow the dog to blink. Blinking will melt the ointment and spread a thin layer evenly over the eye.

Nail Care

The nails of a dog are very similar to our nails. There is a point of dead, thickened skin and an inner core of fleshy tissue that contains the blood and nerve supply, called the *quick*. Anyone who has cut a dog's nail too short knows that it hurt the dog, and it probably bled a lot.

Let's take a closer look at the nail, nail bed and pad. The nail, or claw, is made up of both the continuation of skin epidermis (the dead tip) and the continuation of skin dermis (the quick). The nail grows out of the nail bed, which is the center of the toe. The nail is firmly attached in the nail bed. The pad is the bottom of the toe. It has a black, horny, rough layer of dead epidermis. Beneath that is a pad of fleshy, fatty tissue that is well-vascularized. Anyone who's ever had a dog with a cut pad knows how much they bleed.

In the outdoors, nails are very important for normal walking. Dogs use their nails for traction and tactile feeling. Many dogs nowadays live indoors and walk on hard floors and roads. The nails are still important to these urban dogs, but if they get too long, they can cause a loss of traction. There-fore, dogs who live in places with hard flooring should have their nails trimmed frequently.

Several things can go wrong with nails. We will describe each one in detail.

Bacterial Infections of the Nail Bed (Bacterial Paronychia). The nail bed is prone to injury and abrasions. Small scratches allow opportunistic bacteria to enter the skin and nail bed. Bacteria often grown out of these infections are *Staphylococcus* and *Escherichia coli*. *Staphylococcus* is a common bacterium always present on the skin of dogs. *Escherichia coli* is a bacterium found in feces that gets into the ground. The infection causes inflammation and pain of the skin around the base of the nail. A pus discharge is often present. Treatment is fourfold:

1. Soak the paw in warm water with an antiseptic, such as Epsom salts or Betadine, for five to ten minutes three times daily.

2. Apply topical antibiotic creams or powders.

3. Use oral antibiotics if the infection is deep.

4. As a last resort, if the preceding steps fail, the nail (which is usually loose at this point) can be surgically removed by a veterinarian to allow proper drainage.

Fungal Infection of the Nail Bed (Fungal Paronychia). This is identical to the bacterial paronychia, but the infectious agent is a fungus instead of bacteria. The fungi most often cultured from these infections are *Microsporum* (ringworm fungus) and *Candida*. The look is very similar to the bacterial infection, except the skin is crusty and there may be intense itching. The treatment is very similar to the bacterial infection:

1. Soak the paw in warm water with an antifungal agent such as Betadine for five to ten minutes three times daily.

2. Apply topical antifungal creams.

3. Give oral antifungal drugs.

4. Remove the nail surgically.

Brittle and Cracked Nails. Many dog nails become dry and brittle, especially the longer they get. Superficial cracks and splits are of little consequence. The superficial layer may peel. If the nail crack is deeper, it can go into the quick of the nail bed. This is very painful and can lead to infection. Soaking the nail in warm water and Epsom salts, then applying petroleum jelly, can help. Try to keep the nails short to prevent this condition.

Ingrown Nails. Almost everyone has had an ingrown nail at one time. These are particularly common in toy breed dogs, when the owner doesn't trim the nails often enough. Since canine nails grow in a curved fashion, the point of the nail can curl around and pierce the pad. If left untreated, the nail continues to grow into the pad. Infection ensues shortly thereafter. The owner notices the puppy going lame on the leg. There is usually a bloody discharge and an infectious odor. Once an owner notices the blood on the fur around the nail, he seeks veterinary care. Treatment is simple: The offending nail needs to be cut short and pulled out from the pad. Since this condition is so painful, a local or topical anesthetic is needed to numb the area. Once desensitized, the nail can be cut and removed from the pad. The paw is then soaked in warm antiseptic solutions or Epsom salts three times daily for a week. Oral antibiotics are usually dispensed as well. Dewclaws are prone to being ingrown.

Broken Nails. This is perhaps the worst of the nail ailments. When we say broken, we mean broken off at the base. You can imagine how painful that must be. This occurs when an overgrown nail gets caught and enough torque is applied to break it off at the base. If the nail breaks off cleanly, the fleshy stump of the quick is exposed. This is extremely sensitive and bleeds. At this point, the paw must be soaked in a warm antiseptic solution or Epsom salts three times daily for a week. The vet will often put a bandage on the paw to cover the quick. If the quick continues to bleed, it may need to be chemically cauterized so that the bleeding stops. If the nail doesn't completely break off and is left dangling by a thread, the veterinarian needs to trim off the nail. Since this condition is so painful, a local or topical anesthetic is needed to numb the area. Once desensitized, the nail can be trimmed off. The exposed quick is treated the same way. Antibiotics are often used to prevent infection.

Why Shorter Is Better

Just reading through the descriptions of all the things that can go wrong with nails, you will notice that the majority of them are due to being overgrown.

If you are reluctant to cut your puppy's nails yourself, have your veterinarian or groomer do it as soon as a curved tip grows out. If your dog's nails are clear, you can see the quick *and stay away from it!* If you cut the nail too short, you will cut into the quick, cause undue pain to your dog, and cause a

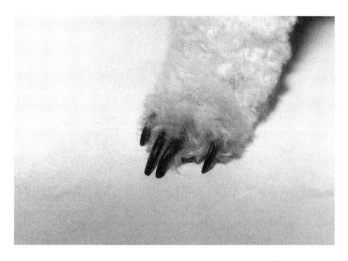

Nails that are too long, like these, are prone to injury, splitting, cracking, breaking off at the base and infection.

moderate amount of bleeding. If the nails are black, you won't be able to see the quick, which makes cutting the nails much more difficult. Either way, follow the next steps or have a professional cut the nails. *Dogs have very good memories. If you cut their nails too short and make them bleed, the dogs may never let you or anyone else try again.*

It's a good idea for any new puppy owner to learn how to cut his or her puppy's nails. Look over these guidelines and decide whether you should attempt it:

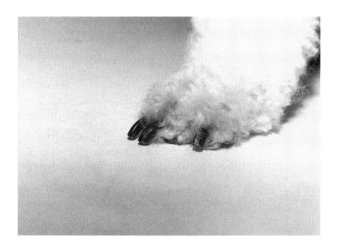

Properly trimmed nails.

- Front nails grow longer and wear slower than hind nails. Therefore, concentrate on the front nails. The average dog needs its nails trimmed every two months.

- Dewclaws are the small nails halfway between the toes and the wrist (on the front legs) and the toes and the hock (on the hind legs). They are not used for walking and usually don't wear down at all. This means they tend to grow long and curl. Don't forget to trim them. Some breeds, like the Great Pyrenees, have double declaws— so don't miss any.

- Dogs that walk on roads, concrete, sidewalks and gravel tend to wear down their nails much faster than dogs that walk only on lawns, dirt, carpeting or hardwood flooring. In fact, dogs that regularly wear down their nails may not need them trimmed.

- Get your puppy used to nail clipping early. Start trimming its nails at eight to ten weeks of age. Handle the paws every day to get your puppy used to people touching its paws. Dogs naturally don't like it, but they can learn to accept it. Be gentle, and hold each toe in your fingers. Count to ten (that's about how long it'll take you to cut the nail). It may take a week of practice before you actually attempt to cut one.

- If your puppy gets aggressive—for example, it growls and tries to bite while you attempt to cut its nails—stop and consult a professional.

Cutting the Nails

There are two basic type of nail cutters: the guillotine-style cutters and the large nail trimmers. Amateurs should use the guillotine-style cutters; they are easier to maneuver and make it harder to cut the nail short. The large trimmers are designed for large nails and can double as a tree pruner; in other words, only someone experienced should use them.

1. Hold the paw with your left hand if you're right-handed or with your right hand if you're left-handed.

2. Cut the nail parallel to the floor, and only cut off the tip of the nail. Start cutting where the tip begins to curve. If the nail is clear and you can see the quick, leave at least one-quarter inch of nail beyond the quick.

3. Cut each nail slowly and carefully. Don't rush this. You may only get a few nails done at one time.

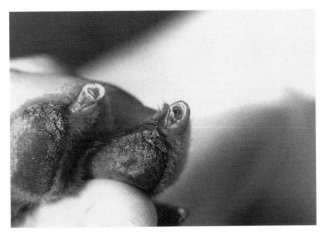

Nails cut so short the quick is exposed, like these, are very painful to the dog.

4. If the puppy is kicking and struggling, don't attempt it. That's how accidents happen.

5. If the nail is left sharp from the cutting, you can use a nail file to round off the end.

What do you do if by accident you cut a nail short? There are commercial products you can buy at pet stores that stop the bleeding. They come in powders and lotions. They all tend to sting like a styptic pencil does. If you don't have one of these in the house, plunge the bleeding end of the nail into a bar of soap. This will work just as well.

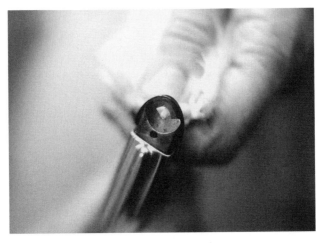

Amateurs should use guillotine-style clippers like these because they're easier to maneuver.

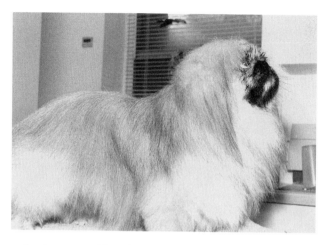

This Pekingese is a long-coated breed with a downy undercoat and a longer, coarser overcoat.

Coat Care

Dogs have several different types of coats. We all think of dog fur as hair. It is, but it's very different from our own. A dog's hair follicles, out of which hair grows, are much closer together, so the hair grows in very dense. In most breeds, the "coat" is really made up of two layers: the overcoat and the undercoat.

Overcoat. These are the longer, coarser hairs—the protective layer. The overcoat protects against sun, water, thorns and brush, animal bites and heat. The oils that the dog's skin secretes keep this layer waterproof. This is more apparent in some breeds. For instance, the Labrador Retriever is a bird dog and has an oily overcoat. The water rolls off the back of a Lab like it rolls off a duck.

Undercoat. This coat is the underneath layer and is made up of finer and shorter hairs. Some people refer to this coat as the *downy* layer. In fact, the undercoat is an insulating layer. Some breeds have more of this layer than others. Taking our Labrador as an example, it has very little undercoat compared to a Chow Chow or a Keeshond.

There are many different varieties of texture of coats as well. Breeds are distinguished as separate breeds based on the texture of their coat. Smooth- and rough-coated Collies are examples. Following is a partial listing of coat varieties:

Lengths: Ultra-Short, Short, Medium, Long

Thicknesses: Fine, Coarse

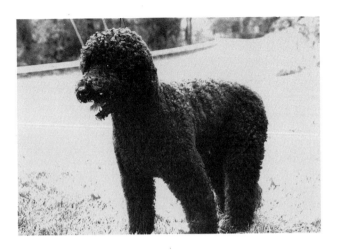

A Portuguese Water Dog, shown here, is a curly-coated breed.

Textures: Smooth, Rough, Flat, Wirehaired, Curly, Wavy, Silky, Woolly, Marcel, Corded, Soft

Colors: Dogs' coats come in many different colors, too, with only a few choices available in each breed. Most colors, and their variations, are listed here:

Whites: White, Cream

Tans: Buff, Champagne, Fawn, Lemon, Mustard, Tan, Tawny, Wheaten, Yellow

Blacks and Browns: Black, Brown, Chocolate, Liver, Mocha, Seal

Silvers and Grays: Gray, Grizzle (blue-gray), Pepper, Salt and Pepper, Silver

Reds: Apricot, Chestnut, Golden, Mahogany, Red, Rust

Blues: Blue, Blue Merle (blue marbling)

Multiple colors: Brindle (black stripes on chestnut background), Harlequin (white base color with patches of blue or black), Pinto (two main colors), Sable (fawn color with black tips) and Tricolor (three colors)

Breeders and groomers use many terms when describing coat types. Many of these terms are used only by dog enthusiasts and in show circles, but it doesn't hurt to be familiar with them.

Glossary of Coat Terms

Apron. The longer fur on the chest.

ASCOB Stands for "Any Solid Color Other than Black."

Belton. A pattern in setters in which two colors, one light and one dark, are mottled together.

Double-coated. A breed that has an overcoat and an undercoat (most breeds).

Feathers and Fringe. Long hairs on the front and hind legs, behind ears and on tail.

Furnishings. Same as feathers and fringe.

Horsecoat. An ultra-short coat that is bristle-like. Seen in the Chinese SharPei.

Parti-color. Two or more colors in well-defined patches.

Penciled. Fine black striping on the toes.

Pily. Intertwining of two hair types.

Points. The color on the face, eyebrows, ears, legs and tail.

Ruff. The mane, or thick coat around the neck.

Saddle. A dark patch covering the back.

Single-coated. Breeds with only an overcoat (such as the Maltese).

Spotted. Having many randomly spaced spots.

Skirt. The long hairs hanging down from the sides and flanks that form a ruffle.

Ticked. Small specks of dark hairs on a white background.

Shedding. All dogs shed to some degree. There are three classes of shedding: light shedders, normal shedders and heavy shedders. Shedding is the turning over of the coat based on photoperiod (hours of light in a day) and seasons. A thicker coat will grow in for the winter, and the shedding will be less. In the spring, the shedding season starts, and the dog will lose much of the undercoat that grew in during the winter. Breeders call this sudden onset of shedding *blowing coat*. Other reasons why dogs can suddenly drop a lot of hair are listed the following page:

- Short-term, excessive nervousness or excitement (like being at the vet's office or the groomers')

- Long-term stress (like being at a boarding kennel)

- Malnutrition, vitamin and mineral deficiencies

- Hormonal changes in females: spaying, heat cycles, pregnancy, false pregnancy

- Allergies and allergic dermatitis

- Parasites: mites and mange, fleas, lice

- Genetic causes: patterned baldness, congenital alopecia

- Diseases: dermatitis, pyoderma, hot spots, ringworm, autoimmune diseases, hypothyroidism, Cushing's disease

Basic Home Grooming

Let's start by making this very clear: Some breeds *require* regular professional grooming. In many states, groomers are certified and have gone to school to learn their trade. Here is a partial list of these breeds:

Afghan Hound
Airedale Terrier
Akita
Alaskan Malamute
Australian Shepherd
Bearded Collie
Bedlington Terrier
Belgian Sheepdog
Belgian Tervuren
Bernese Mountain
  Dog
Bichon Frise
Borzoi
Bouvier des Flandres
Briard
Brussels Griffon
Cairn Terrier
Chow Chow
Cocker Spaniel
Collie (Rough)
Dandie Dinmont
  Terrier

English Springer
  Spaniel
Great Pyrenees
Irish Terrier
Irish Water Spaniel
Keeshond
Kerry Blue Terrier
Komodor
Kuvasz
Lakeland Terrier
Lhasa Apso
Maltese
Newfoundland
Norwegian Elkhound
Old English Sheepdog
Otterhound
Pekingese
Pomeranian
Poodle, all varieties
Portuguese Water
  Dog
Puli

Saint Bernard
Saluki
Samoyed
Schnauzer, all sizes
Scottish Terrier
Sealyham Terrier
Shetland Sheepdog
Shih Tzu
Silky Terrier
Skye Terrier
Soft Coated Wheaten
  Terrier
Tibetan Terrier
Welsh Springer
  Spaniel
Welsh Terrier
West Highland
  White Terrier
Wire Fox Terrier
Yorkshire Terrier

The breeds on this list are either very difficult to groom or their coats are so thick and coarse that professional equipment is required to get through them. Some breeds have such intricate grooming patterns that the average owner could not follow them. After all, you wouldn't want your Poodle to come out looking like a julienned french fry!

Breeds that aren't on this list, including many of the short-coated breeds, can be groomed at home. If a breed can be put in a tub, towel dried and combed out without too much fuss, then it's considered an easily groomed breed. Examples are the Labrador Retriever, Beagle, Pug and Great Dane.

Tools of the Trade

Before you can get started with basic grooming at home, you need to know what tools are available and which one you use for what job. Here are some guidelines to follow:

Wire Slicker Brush. This is the most common brush people buy for their dog. It has angled wires to brush the coat and is designed to get through medium to short coats. It doesn't detangle mats. If used on a dense coat, it tends to skim over the surface of the coat, not really doing anything.

Universal Wire Brush. This is very similar to the slicker brush but is stronger and can work through some mats. This is a popular tool for brushing dogs.

Combs. Several different combs are on the market. Most are stainless steel, and some are Teflon-coated. They come in different tooth widths, from fine to medium to coarse. Combs are best at getting out mats or teasing snarls. Combs with ultrafine teeth are called *flea combs*. They are used to trap and comb out adult fleas from the coats of dogs and cats.

Rakes. These are great for pulling out dead undercoat from a densely coated dog. Make sure you get the ones with rounded teeth; otherwise you could scrape the puppy's skin. These must be used gently.

Shedding Blade. This looks like a bowed saw blade with saw teeth. It is used to pull out dead overcoat. You must be very careful with this tool: Too much pressure will cause scrapes and abrasions to the skin.

Mat Comb. This should be used only by an experienced professional. It's a comb with wide razor-sharp teeth for cutting into mats.

Scissors. Scissors are used to cut hair. High-quality scissors can cut through matted hair like butter. They must be kept sharp and clean to cut well. There are different types of scissors: *straight barber scissors*, which are ideal for trimming hair in a straight line, such as on the legs; *curved barber scissors*, which are ideal for shaping rounded areas such as pom-poms; *thinning shears*, which are special scissors that thin out a dense coat and are also used for blending between two different areas; and *blunt-tipped scissors*, which have rounded tips, making them safer around the face and eyes (they're also great for getting in between toes and inside ears).

Clippers. These are electric shavers that have interchangeable blades. They are used by professionals and experienced amateurs. Clippers can cut through the toughest of mats and can shave as close as a razor.

Shampoos. Shampoos for dogs are similar to those for people, but there are some differences. One of the biggest is the pH level. A dog shampoo is pH balanced for canine hair. A good shampoo will be easy to work with, lather well, smell nice and rinse thoroughly with no residue. Many different types of shampoos are available, from insecticide to medicated. They can contain ingredients to clean, detangle, medicate, reduce itching and flaking, deodorize and whiten. Following is a list of some active ingredients and what they do:

Shampoo Ingredients and Their Actions		
Active Ingredient	**Action**	**Possible Uses**
Tearless Shampoo	Cleaner	general cleaning
Insecticide	kills fleas and ticks	flea infestation
Whitener	bleaches fur	bleach out tear stains
Deodorizer	inactivates odors	skunk bath
Citrus Oils	kills fleas and deodorizes	general cleaner, fleas
Shampoo and Conditioner	de-tangles	mildly tangled dogs
Colloidal Oatmeal	anti-itch	allergic dermatitis
Coal Tar and Sulfur	reduces itch and flaking	seborrhea
Herbal and Aloe Vera	luster	before a show

Other Grooming Aids. Other products can help you groom your new puppy at home. They can detangle mats, deodorize and freshen your puppy's hair, and generally make your job easier.

Grooming Your Dog

Before getting down to business, do a few preparatory steps:

1. Clean the ears with an ear cleaner and cotton, as described earlier in this chapter.

2. Place cotton in the puppy's ears to keep water out during the bath.

Step 1: Brushing and Combing. Before the water touches your dog, you have to brush out the coat *thoroughly*. Matted hair turns into cement when it gets wet (a slight exaggeration, but you get the idea). The rule is that you should spend more time brushing and combing out the coat than you do bathing the puppy. Do specific areas one at a time; i.e., do each leg individually, then work on the tail. Cover the entire body in a logical fashion so that you don't miss any areas. Use your brush first; then go over the coat again with the comb, and end with another brushing. This will really get all the snags and tangles out. Don't miss those hard-to-get areas, like under the tail, behind the ears and between the hind legs. When you're finished brushing the coat, it should have a luster, feel soft and be free of most of the dead hair. Brushing spreads the natural oils of the coat. In fact, a brush-out will suffice to clean the dog's coat most of the time, but bathing is needed occasionally.

Step 2: The Bath. Once the brush-out is done, it's time for the bath. If done indoors, using the bathtub is best. Some people use the garden hose outside, weather permitting. Using warm water, completely wet the coat, starting at the head, and work your way down to the tail. Then apply the shampoo, again starting at the head. Work up a good lather. Use your fingers to work the lather thoroughly into the coat. Rinsing is next. Use plenty of warm water. Rinse until you can't feel any soapy residue. When finished, wring the water out of the coat with your fingers. At this point, the dog usually shakes the excess water all over you, and you both get a bath!

Step 3: Drying. After squeezing the water out of the coat, use a thick cotton towel to towel-dry the coat. You may need two or three towels for a large, long-coated breed. If you have a blow dryer, you can use it on the low setting, never closer than twelve inches from the skin. In warm weather, you can skip the blow drying.

Step 4: Final Brush-Out. The final step in the process is to brush the coat out again. Now your dog is fresh and clean. Wow, what a difference!

How often should you groom and bathe your puppy? It's a good idea to brush your puppy every day. Go over the entire body, looking for sore spots or scratches, checking toenails, keeping ears and eyes clean and brushing teeth. If your puppy gets dirty easily, you can bathe it as often as every couple of weeks. Just be careful not to overbathe, as this can dry out the coat. Most people with breeds that require professional grooming have it done every six to eight weeks.

Feeding and Nutrition

The old saying "You are what you eat" is especially true in animals. If just one nutrient is out of proportion or deficient, disease will result. We will cover some of the most common nutritional deficiencies later in the chapter. But in fact, the average American dog eats a more balanced and complete diet than the average American person. This is because extensive research has gone into what constitutes a dog's daily requirements of the food groups, vitamins and minerals. A standardized minimum level is determined for each and every nutrient, as stated by the National Academy of Sciences Nutrient Requirements (NRC) for dogs. When a commercial dog food claims to be "complete and balanced," it meets these daily requirements. This standard has been set up by the AAFCO (Association of American Feed Control Officials).

What Is a Nutrient?

Nutrients are the substances required to sustain life:

The Six Nutrients	
Nutrient	Function
Water	Large quantities of water are needed daily to prevent dehydration and for normal bodily function.
Proteins	Proteins are the building blocks of muscle, connective tissue, enzymes and hormones.

continues

The Six Nutrients (*continued*)	
Nutrient	**Function**
Carbohydrates	These are sources of energy, sugars and fiber for normal digestion.
Fats	Fats are essential for the absorption of fat-soluble vitamins; to provide storage for energy in times of fasting; to provide fatty acids for the coat; and to make food more palatable.
Vitamins	Vitamins are needed in small quantities for bodily functions.
Minerals	Minerals are needed for strong bone, cellular function and cell stability.

Let's look at each group a little more closely. This will give you an idea of why these nutrients are so important in the diet.

Water

Water is the single most important nutrient. Life can continue for weeks without nutrients in the food groups, but without water, clinical dehydration occurs within days. Severe dehydration is terminal. There are two ways to get water naturally: by drinking and by consuming water in foods. The normal daily water intake for a dog at rest (not exercising) and in an ambient temperature of 65°F is *one ounce per pound of body weight.*

Think of it: For a fifty-pound dog, that's fifty ounces of water, or slightly more than six cups of water a day—for just sitting there. Now get the dog walking, playing, or barking, and this number may go up to $1^1/_2$ ounces. Now how about in the summer with temperatures above 80°F? This figure could go as high as 2 to $2^1/_2$ ounces. The fact is that proper water intake is not even this simple to calculate. Smaller dogs actually require more water, and the large dogs may require less. Use the following chart.

Water Requirements for Dogs	
Size	**Ounces/pound of water daily**
Toy Breeds	1.7
Small to Medium Breeds	1
Large Breeds	.83
Giant Breeds	.7

Most dogs self-regulate their water intake. They sense their body dehydrating, so they seek water. Therefore, water should always be available. *Puppies require a lot of water, and restricting it can put your puppy at risk of dehydrating. The only time water can be safely withheld is at night.*

Proteins

Proteins are the building blocks of muscle and connective tissues. Dogs get their protein in their diet, usually from animal-based ingredients and certain bean products. Proteins are digested and broken down into amino acids. These are small molecules used in the production of muscle fibers, hormones and enzymes. There are twenty-two different amino acids. Some can be manufactured by the dog's liver; others must be found in their diet. These indispensable amino acids are called *essential amino acids.*

We grade proteins as either low or high quality. High-quality proteins are ones that meet three requirements. The first is that the proteins have a high *biologic* value, which is the percent that is absorbed and utilized by the body. Poor-quality proteins are not retained by the body and are excreted in the urine. The second feature of a high-quality protein is that it contains many *essential amino acids.* The third factor is *digestibility*, which means that the protein is actually digested and doesn't just pass out in the feces. A good percentage of digestibility is 80 percent in dry foods, 90 percent in canned.

High-quality proteins can be found in animal source foods: beef, lamb and poultry, for example. Meat by-products and vegetable sources (such as soybeans) are not as good. The quality of the protein becomes more important when there is a deficiency of it in the diet. The minimum protein level in a puppy's diet should be around 25 percent. Some foods boast "high protein" levels as high as 30 percent. You can be sure that some of this protein will be wasted and excreted in the urine. In order for the body to utilize the most protein from the food as it can, there has to be a certain amount of calories in the food. In other words, there may be lots of high-quality protein in the diet, but if there aren't enough high-energy calories, the body can't use the protein. Also, protein excreted in the urine has to be filtered through the kidneys. All this excess filtering is very stressful to the kidneys. *Therefore, when it comes to protein, more isn't necessarily better. Stick to a diet that has high-quality protein which is 25 percent on a dry basis (versus wet food).*

Carbohydrates

Ah, do we all love carbohydrates. This is the group of nutrients that contains *starches*, *sugars* and *fiber.* Bread, pasta, cereal, rice, potatoes, vegetables, biscuits, cookies and grains are all carbohydrates. Carbohydrates supply the majority of energy in a dog's diet. If too many carbohydrates are eaten, they don't get excreted out of the body like protein. They get stored as fat, a future energy source. The body needs carbohydrates to utilize proteins. Too many lead to obesity. There are three basic types of carbohydrates: *simple, complex* and *dietary fiber. Simple carbohydrates* are the sugars. Certain sugars can be absorbed directly from the food without digestion, like glucose; others need to be broken down to be absorbed, like the fruit sugar, fructose. *Complex carbohydrates* are found in whole grains, fruits and vegetables. These are the foods that give sustained energy. *Dietary fibers* are the nondigestible carbohydrates that aid in normal digestion. These fibers keep the food and stool moving through the intestines. Too many fiber-rich foods will lead to diarrhea because they move through the system too quickly. *There must be a balance between sugars and fiber for proper digestion. Fiber should be between 3 to 4 percent of the diet on a dry basis (versus wet food).*

Fats

There has been a lot of publicity about fats lately, most of it bad. In people, diets high in fat, especially saturated fat, have been linked to heart disease, obesity and certain types of cancer. Saturated fats are found in animal fats, hydrogenated vegetable oils and tropical oils, such as palm seed and coconut oils. Unsaturated fats found in unprocessed vegetable oils seem to be the healthiest ones.

Having said that, let me now enumerate the good things fats and oils do. First, fats are needed in the diet to allow absorption of fat-soluble vitamins (namely A, D, E and K). Second, fats contain essential fatty acids needed for the synthesis of cell membranes and hormones, and for a healthy coat and skin. Deficiencies of fatty acids lead to skin and coat problems, as will be discussed later. Third, fats make foods *palatable,* meaning tasty. Studies have shown that people find fatty foods "comforting," while animals find them appetizing. Fourth, fats are easily digested and are stored as a quickly mobilized energy source—namely, fat. In other words, if a diet rich in fats and oils is eaten regularly, the excess fats will end up as fatty deposits. We all know this to be true (can you pinch an inch?).

Premium puppy foods generally are not less than 20 percent fat on a dry basis (versus wet food), due to the high demand for fats in this age group.

Unfortunately, in most commercially available dog foods, the fat added needs to be preserved to keep it from *oxidizing,* or going rancid. Rancid fat is harmful if eaten. This means that the manufacturer needs to add preservatives in order to allow a long shelflife of the food.

Vitamins

Do you take vitamins? We find that people who take vitamins themselves usually give them to their pets. The question is, Do you need to give vitamins to your puppy? The answer is a bit complicated. Let's start by saying that most of the commercial dog foods on the market are "complete and balanced." This means they contain the daily requirements for all nutrients, including vitamins and minerals, which implies that no supplementation is needed. This is true for the average dog. If, however, you have a puppy that is very athletic or works every day, then your puppy will have a higher requirement for these nutrients. Before we get into what and how much to supplement, let's look into what vitamins are used to fortify dog foods, and what they do.

There are two groups of vitamins: water-soluble and fat-soluble. Water-soluble vitamins (B_1, B_2, niacin, folic acid, biotin, B_6, B_{12}, C) can dissolve in water and are filtered through the kidneys when there is an excess of them in the body. Fat-soluble vitamins (A, D, E, K) are not dissolvable in water and end up in places where fats congregate, such as the liver, skin and blood. Here is a table of the common vitamins and what they do:

Vitamins		
Vitamin	**Natural Source**	**Function**
A	orange vegetables	needed for sight, skin texture
D	dairy foods	needed for strong bone, teeth, calcium
E	oils and fats	Antioxidant to maintain fats, muscle
K	digestive by-products	needed for blood clotting
B_1, B_2, Niacin, Folic Acid, Biotin, B_6, B_{12}	whole grains, eggs, oils	stimulates appetite, needed for normal cellular function
C	citrus fruits, vegetables	maintains immune system, prevents scurvy

Vitamin deficiencies will be covered later in this chapter. Most experts agree that it is better to get vitamins from natural sources than from vitamin tablets. The experts believe that such vitamins are more available and better absorbed (better bioavailability).

Minerals

Minerals, sometimes called "ash," are needed in minute quantities to sustain life. They are the fundamental building blocks of bone and teeth, and are needed for cellular functions. Minerals are also salts, which are crucial in the maintenance of tissues and cells. The minerals needed in fairly large amounts in the diet are calcium, iron, phosphorus, potassium, sodium and zinc. The minerals needed in trace amounts from the diet are copper, iodine, magnesium, manganese and selenium.

Minerals are basically obtained from foods, water and salts. Certain foods are high in minerals; for example, dark green leafy vegetables have a lot of calcium. The following chart shows where some of these minerals come from:

Minerals		
Mineral	Natural Source	Function
Calcium	green leafy vegetables	strong bones and teeth, cellular function
Copper	nuts and beans	needed for blood cells, nerves and bone
Iodine	seafood, kelp	needed for normal thyroid function
Iron	meats	oxygen transport of red blood cells
Magnesium	dairy foods, fish, grain	needed for bone, muscle, heart function
Phosphorus	grains, nuts, dairy	bone, teeth, kidney function
Potassium	dairy, fish, meats, fruit	nerves, heart rhythm, kidney function
Selenium	nuts, grains	fat preservation, anti-oxidant
Sodium	most foods	body water balance, all nerve functions
Zinc	seafood, meats, eggs	healthy skin and coat

Even though some of these minerals are only required in minute amounts, without them there would be illness. Mineral deficiencies are covered at the end of this chapter.

Are All Dog Foods Alike?

The simple answer is "No." Most commercially available foods are "complete and balanced," but the similarity ends there. As mentioned previously, there are differences in the quality of the ingredients used. This is especially true for protein. Here are some questions to ask yourself before buying dog food:

- Should I buy a dry or canned food; which is better for my puppy?
- Is my puppy under six months old or between six months and one year old?
- Is my puppy very active or basically sedentary?
- Will my puppy eat dry food, or have I already spoiled him with canned food?
- Is my puppy a toy, medium to large or giant breed?
- Will I be expecting maximum performance from him during sport, work or exercise?
- Is stool volume a concern to me?
- Has my puppy shown an allergy to any main ingredient?
- Does my puppy have a flatulence problem?
- Can I afford the expensive premium foods?
- Should I buy puppy food at a pet store or a grocery store?

The next step is to take a close look at the different types of dog foods. There are three forms of dog food: dry (kibble or expanded), canned and semimoist foods. Most veterinarians recommend feeding dry food, which is generally more nutritious and better balanced by virtue of being mostly food and not water like the canned foods (canned foods are close to 75 percent water). Also, as mentioned earlier in this chapter, dry foods are better for maintaining healthy teeth and gums than are canned foods, which are more likely to put tartar on the teeth. I recommend keeping the canned food to less than 25 percent of the daily intake by weight, if the owners insist on feeding it. Think of canned food as a treat and not a main staple of the diet. As far as the semimoist foods are concerned, we regard them as the "junk" foods. They're laden with sugars, artificial colors and preservatives, and should be avoided.

The first way to classify dog foods is based on which age group they are formulated for: a puppy, adult or senior (less active). Since this is a puppy book, we'll focus on the puppy foods.

The second way to classify dog foods is by their quality. Here are the basic categories: performance, premium, high-quality, average and economy foods. What these categories are based on is the percentage of protein, fat and fiber in the food, as well as the quality of the main ingredients and whether preservatives or artificial ingredients are used. Generally speaking, performance and premium foods have higher levels of protein and fat, with reduced fiber for a smaller stool. They are also more natural foods with few if any artificial ingredients or preservatives. We have already mentioned that too much protein can be stressful to the kidneys. But that becomes a concern when a dog has spent years consuming a high-protein food. This is not a concern in puppies. Puppies have higher requirements for protein, fat, vitamins and minerals than do adult dogs, except perhaps for lactating bitches or dogs used for intense work or sport.

"Guaranteed Analysis" and Ingredients

How can you tell which foods are considered premium or "high quality"? Read the labels! On each package or can of dog food, there is a label with a "guaranteed analysis" listing. This is a rough measure of how much protein, fat and water (moisture) is in the food on a dry-matter basis (discounting the water). The reason the estimates are rough is because they are listed as "not more than" maximums for water and fiber, and "not less than" minimums for proteins and fat values. I always check for grams of fat per ounce or serving, for example. Here are some guidelines to go by that can give you an idea of what to expect from a premium food.

Guidelines for Guaranteed Analysis in Premium Foods			
Nutrient	Minimum %	Maximum %	Main Ingredient Source
Protein	25	N/A	chicken, chicken by-products, lamb, beef, egg
Fat	15	N/A	chicken fat, beef tallow, lamb fat, vegetable oil
Fiber	N/A	4	ground corn, rice, barley, corn gluten, bran, beet pulp
Water	N/A	10	N/A

N/A—not applicable

The other important thing to read on the food label is the list of ingredients. This is a list of all the ingredients in descending order. In other words, the first ingredient is what there is the most of, and the last one is in the least amount. This is important to know, because if the main protein source is listed third, for example, then you could suspect the food had a low protein content.

What, How Much and When to Feed Your Puppy

Let's start with what to feed your puppy. We just described in detail what to expect from a premium food. Do you have to feed your puppy a premium diet? Well no, you don't. But allow me to make an analogy. Think about how you feel after eating a bag of potato chips and a candy bar. A bit bloated, thirsty and wired? Now think about how you feel after eating a home-cooked meal of chicken, a fresh salad, mashed potatoes and gravy? You'd feel full, but energetic, awake and content. Do you get the point? The better the food, the healthier your puppy will be inside and out: stronger bones and connective tissue, bright eyes, healthy teeth and gums, resilient skin, lustrous coat, high energy, good muscle tone and an even temperament. Do you have to buy the most expensive food on the market? No, get one that meets the requirements as discussed in this chapter. This should be easy to find in a puppy formula. We don't recommend buying bargain food that is mostly corn meal or cereal. Your puppy couldn't possibly thrive on that. As far as where to buy your food, high-quality puppy foods are available at both pet stores and at the grocery store. All you have to do is read the label! *Always feed your puppy a diet formulated for puppies. Adult maintenance foods don't usually have the level of nutrients needed for a growing puppy with a high metabolism.*

How much to feed is the next issue. Most bags and cans of dog food have a chart on the back label that gives feeding instructions. We have found these guidelines often exaggerate how much a puppy will eat at one sitting. You can use the following chart to get a basic idea of how much to feed for both dry and canned foods.

Daily Amounts for Dry and Canned Foods		
Weight in Pounds	Cups[†] per Day of Dry Food	Cans[‡] per Day of Canned Food
1–10	1–1$\frac{1}{2}$	$\frac{1}{2}$–1
11–30	2–2$\frac{1}{2}$	2
31–45	4	2$\frac{1}{2}$
46–60	5–6	3–3$\frac{1}{2}$
61–75	6–7	4–4$\frac{1}{2}$
76–90	7–8	4$\frac{1}{2}$–5
over 100	8–9	5–5$\frac{1}{2}$

†Based on 8 oz. cups. ‡Based on 15 oz. cans.

Please use this chart as a guideline only. Watching weight gains and consulting with your vet are the best ways to determine whether you're overfeeding or underfeeding your puppy.

The last consideration of feeding is when to feed. This is something we are very adamant about. The feeding schedule is very important for housebreaking. You never want to free-choice feed your puppy, meaning the food is in the bowl all the time. If you do, we can almost assure you your efforts to housebreak will be wasted—and your puppy could get quite sick. The reward of a regular feeding schedule is easier housebreaking.

Some of you may be saying, "I thought that dogs only needed to be fed once a day." Most people find that dividing the total daily quantity of food into two equal portions keeps their dog from ever becoming too hungry. Some dogs become nauseous or weak if they go twenty-four hours without eating. This can lead to obsessive behavior and dry heaving. *We find that dogs thrive better with two feedings a day, even as adults.*

Are Table Scraps OK?

Most veterinarians will tell you that feeding table scraps to your puppy is bad for it. Here are some of the reasons why:

- Table scraps put more tartar on the teeth than dog food does.
- They usually are more fattening for a dog than dog food is.
- They may be more difficult to digest than dog food is.
- They will upset the intestinal balance, causing vomiting and diarrhea.
- They only spoil the puppy (who now won't eat his dog food).
- They rarely have the nutrition your puppy needs and gets from dog food.

Having said all that, you may be shocked to find out that the vast majority of new puppy owners do feed table scraps. Why? Perhaps it's that special way the puppy looks at you when you're eating its favorite dish. That little face can be so expressive, can't it? We've all been there. Therefore, if you insist on feeding your puppy table scraps from your plate, follow these guidelines:

Feeding Schedule		
Age	Feedings per Day	Snacks Allowed
6 weeks to 3 months	4	yes, often
3 months to 6 months	3	yes, often
6 months to 1 year	2	yes, but occasional
after 1 year	2	try to limit between-meal snacks

Nutritional Supplements

Many people ask whether they should give their puppy vitamins or other supplements. The answer is: If you're feeding one of the premium foods that meet the requirements listed earlier in this chapter, no supplementation is needed. Many people are tempted to supplement the diets of large or giant breeds to enhance their rate of weight gain and encourage them to be bigger, faster. This is a bad idea, especially because these breeds are prone to developmental problems if they grow too fast. Such a disorder is called *panosteitis*; some people refer to it as "growing pains." This condition is covered in detail under "Musculoskeletal Diseases" in Chapter 6. Others feel that overfeeding and oversupplementing can predispose a puppy to hip dysplasia. *What we want to emphasize here is that unless your puppy is unusually active or used for sport or work, a balanced premium diet is likely to be all it will need.*

Some owners, however, insist on feeding supplements. Following is a list of some nutritional supplements added to diets:

- Protein as meat or soybean, for energy and a lustrous coat
- Fat as beef or poultry tallow, for added warmth in dogs subjected to cold climates
- Calcium in the form of bone meal or crushed oyster shells, for strong bones
- Phosphorus in combination with calcium, to keep a 1.4:1 ratio
- Simple sugars like glucose, sucrose and dextrose, as ready energy sources
- Vitamins (the most common being E, $B_{1,2,6,12}$, A and D
- Trace minerals such as copper, zinc, iron, manganese, iodine, potassium and cobalt
- Fatty acids in fish oils, for coat and skin

These supplements can be found in chewable daily vitamins, in liquid vitamins or in their natural sources. People who study nutrition make their own formulas by combining natural ingredients. They feel that the nutrient is more available in a natural source than in a processed purified supplement. Natural sources can include wheat germ oil (vitamin E); cod liver oil (fatty acids, vitamins A and D); bone meal (calcium and phosphorus); bananas (potassium); brewer's yeast (B vitamins); kelp (trace minerals); green, leafy vegetables (calcium and vitamin C); eggs (protein); dairy foods such as yogurt, cottage cheese and evaporated milk (protein, calcium, vitamin D); and beans (protein).

Do's	Dont's
• only feed your puppy scraps you'd eat yourself	• never treat your puppy like a garbage disposal
• stick to chicken, beef, lamb or turkey—other meats can be difficult to digest	• stay away from pork, veal, venison, duck and other gamey meats as they are too fatty
• vegetables are OK if they're cooked	• stay away from raw vegetables except carrots
• rice, potato and plain pasta are satisfactory carbohydrates	• don't feed pastas with sauce or gravy
• wholesome foods like cottage cheese baby food, bread, cheese and yogurt are good in small quantities	• never feed processed foods like potato chips, crackers, pretzels, canned nuts or other salty foods
• dogs may eat small pieces of fruits, including canned fruit	• dogs should never be given candy—especially chocolate, which is toxic to them
• table food should only be a treat once in a while, if at all	• never feed leftover Chinese food, pizza, Mexican or other spicy foods unless you're willing to clean up the mess when it backfires

Nutritional Deficiencies

Now that you know all the right things to feed your puppy, when to feed, what supplements to use if desired, and what not to feed, let's look at what can happen if there is a deficiency of an individual nutrient. The chart on page 155 lists some of the commonly seen nutrient deficiencies and their symptoms.

Spaying and Neutering

Many people use the term "fix" to describe making their dog unbreedable. The actual terminology is *spay* for a female and *neuter* for a male. The typical time for neutering or spaying is when the puppy is six months old. This age is chosen for the following reasons:

> **For a bitch:** Since most bitches don't start coming into heat until this age, you are preventing them from going into their first heat cycle. As you will see a little later in the chapter, spaying has definite benefits in preventing certain types of cancer. It also eliminates the risk of unwanted pregnancy.

Nutrient Deficiencies	
Nutrient	**Deficiency Symptoms**
Protein	dull, brittle coat; low energy; muscle atrophy; swelling of legs
Carbohydrates/Fiber	low energy, hypoglycemia, poor digestion, constipation
Fats/Fatty Acids	dry coat, flaky skin, dermatitis, pansteatitis
Water	dehydration, dry gums, weight loss
Vitamin	**Deficiency Symptoms**
A	poor skin, dull coat, retinal degeneration and blindness
$B_{1,2,6,12}$	weight loss, poor appetite, poor digestion, convulsions, anemia, hindquarter weakness, neck contortion
C	decreased immune system, scurvy
D	poor bone and teeth formation, rickets
E	poor muscle contractions, pansteatitis of fat
K	increased clotting time with excess bleeding, hemophilia
Mineral	**Deficiency Symptoms**
Calcium	poor bone formation, skeletal deformities
Copper	anemia, change of color of fur
Iodine	hypothyroidism, goiter
Iron	anemia
Magnesium	bone and joint deformities, neurological symptoms
Manganese	deformed joints and tendons
Phosphorus	crazed appetite, poor bone formation, skeletal deformities
Potassium	neurological weakness, heart arrhythmia
Selenium	muscle degeneration
Sodium	excess urination, dehydration, salt craving
Zinc	seborrhea, poor flaky coat, baldness

For a dog: Most male dogs don't yet reach puberty by six months of age. Neutering them at this age prevents the male behaviors from developing. For example, he will probably never lift his leg to urinate. Most of the male physical characteristics are developed by this time, so neutering doesn't stunt their growth.

We will describe each procedure in more detail. Please keep in mind that both procedures are surgical, require general anesthesia, have a recuperation period of a couple of weeks and must be performed by a veterinary surgeon.

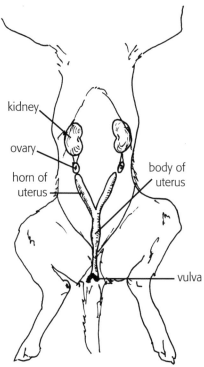

Normal female anatomy before spaying.

Spaying

The spay procedure is a surgical ovariohysterectomy. What this means is that both ovaries and the body of the uterus are surgically removed. To fully understand this procedure, you must first know what these organs do and where they are.

Ovaries. The ovaries are the female gonads. They are suspended from the kidney by a ligament. They manufacture the eggs, which are released during the *estrus*, or "heat" cycle. Most puppy bitches have their first heat cycle at about six to eight months of age (earlier in the larger breeds, later in the toys). Most bitches that have normal cycles will be in heat every six months. During heat, the *vulva* (opening of the vagina) swells, and there is a bloody discharge. The average heat cycle lasts two to three weeks. During this time, the ovaries release the eggs, a process called *ovulation*. Within two to six days after ovulation, the bitch is fertile. This means she will accept a male for breeding, and fertilization of the eggs with the male's sperm is possible. The ovaries are also where the female hormone *estrogen* is secreted. Estrogen is needed for proper development of the female reproductive tract and for the commencement of estrus. Without the ovaries, there are no eggs and virtually no estrogen hormone. The result is no heat cycles and an infertile bitch.

Uterus. The uterus is the tubular organ that holds the developing fetuses during pregnancy. Another name for the uterus is *womb*. In the bitch, it has a "Y" shape, with two horns and a body. The uterus is connected to the vagina by the *cervix*, a sphincter that opens and closes passage into the uterus. When closed, the cervix keeps anything from entering the uterus. When open, it allows sperm to enter (during breeding) or fetuses to exit (during whelping). Without a uterus and a cervix, a dog cannot become pregnant.

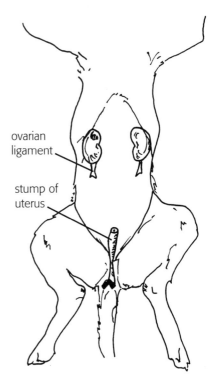

Female anatomy after spaying.

You may be asking yourself why you would want to have your female puppy's uterus and ovaries removed. The most obvious advantage is that she won't go into heat, so she can't breed or get pregnant. The other advantages—and disadvantages—are summarized here.

Advantages of spaying:

- No more messy heat cycles.
- No chance of breeding or unwanted pregnancy.
- You avoid the behavioral changes (restlessness, aggression, roaming and whining) during heat cycles.
- The lack of estrogen hormone prevents breast cancer later in life. Dogs spayed before their second heat cycle have a 95 percent reduction in mammary carcinoma, as compared to intact bitches.
- No chance of ovarian, uterine or cervical cancer.
- You're doing your part in preventing the surplus of unwanted puppies.

Disadvantages of spaying:

- Weight gain is common after spaying, as the base metabolism is lower.
- You cannot ever breed or show a spayed bitch.
- Some people notice a reduction in activity after spaying.
- The risks of the anesthesia and surgery in general are low, but ask your vet whether there are any special considerations regarding your puppy.

Neutering

Neutering is a euphemism for castration. When a male dog is neutered, the two testicles are surgically removed, leaving an empty scrotum. Following is a brief description of the male parts affected by neutering.

> **Testicles.** The testicles are the male gonads, which manufacture sperm cells. Within the testicles are tubules (called *seminiferous tubules*) that produce the sperm cells. The mature sperm cells are stored in a storage sack at the base of the testicle called the *epididymis*. During ejaculation, sperm travels from the testicle up the tube that leads into the abdomen (called the *spermatic cord*) and through the penis (via the *urethra*). The testicle is where the hormone *testosterone* is produced. This hormone is responsible for male sexual characteristics, sexual performance, male physical characteristics, muscle size and male behavior. Testosterone hormone is eliminated when the testicles are removed by neutering.
>
> **Scrotum.** The testicles are housed in a thin-skinned pouch called the *scrotum*, which is a protective as well as a temperature-controlling device. Since sperm production is best at an optimum temperature of about 95°F, the scrotum shrinks in the cold weather to draw the testicles closer to the body for warmth. Conversely, in warm temperatures, the scrotum relaxes, allowing the testicles to sag farther away from the body to keep cool. The scrotum is left intact in neutering.
>
> **Prostate Gland.** The prostate is a walnut-shaped organ that sits at the base of the urinary bladder. The tube that carries urine and sperm runs through the middle of the prostate. The gland secretes fluid during an ejaculation, which aids the sperm's mobility. The prostate is dependent on testosterone to maintain its size and function. Without this hormone, the prostate shrivels up to a small nonfunctioning nub. You may be wondering why you should get your dog neutered. The answer

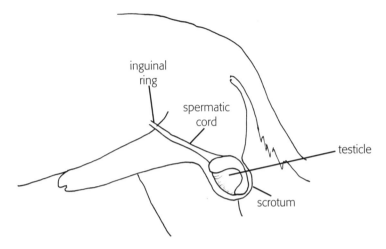

Normal male anatomy before neutering.

is that many people find male behavior undesirable in a house pet. Following is a summary of advantages and disadvantages.

Advantages of Neutering:

- Once the testicles are removed, the testosterone hormone disappears and with it the male behavior many people find objectionable, such as lifting of the hind leg to urinate and "mark" territory, male aggression, male dominance and territorial behavior, roaming to find a mate and mounting of objects and people.
- Testicular cancer is prevented.
- All prostatic diseases such as cancer, prostatic enlargement and prostatitis (infection of the prostate) are prevented.
- Most people find a neutered male a better house pet, especially if they have young children.
- You're doing your part in preventing the surplus of unwanted puppies.

Disadvantages of Neutering:

- Weight gain is common after neutering, as the base metabolism is lower.
- You cannot ever breed or show a neutered dog.
- Some people notice a reduction in activity after neutering. This is a problem if your puppy is used for work, sport or protection.
- The risks of the anesthesia and surgery in general are low, but ask your vet whether there are any special considerations regarding your puppy.

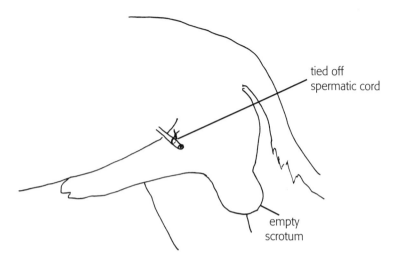

tied off
spermatic cord

empty
scrotum

Male anatomy after neutering.

Cryptorchids, a Special Consideration

As defined in Chapter 1, under "Congenital and Inherited Defects," cryptorchidism is when only one testicle makes it down into the scrotum, leaving the other in the abdomen, or hungup in the *inguinal ring*, the opening where the testicle makes its descent. This problem is genetic. Most puppies that haven't "dropped" both testicles by the time they're four to five months old, won't. This is a problem when it comes time to neuter the dog. You cannot just remove the one testicle that has descended into the scrotum. If the surgeon leaves the internal testicle, testosterone levels will still be sufficient to maintain all the male behavior, and the dog could still breed a bitch in heat. Since this problem is inherited, these dogs should be neutered so that they cannot propagate this defect by breeding. The other reason you should have your cryptorchid dog neutered is because studies have shown that the internal testicle is much more likely to become cancerous later in life than the external one in the scrotum. This is because of the constant higher temperatures inside the abdomen.

Since both testicles of a cryptorchid dog have to be removed, the surgeon has to find the other one. You might think that should be easy. The fact is that the internal testicle can be anywhere in the abdomen or inguinal ring. It is usually small and immature, making it even harder to find. And, to complicate things, some puppies are born with only one testicle—although that's very rare. Therefore, the surgery to neuter a cryptorchid dog is involved and lengthy; it is aptly called an *exploratory* surgery. If the surgeon is lucky, the underdeveloped testicle will be hiding right at the opening of the inguinal ring. I have found testicles in various places, such as under the urinary bladder, adjacent to the prostate gland, under a kidney and sitting just in front of the inner inguinal ring.

It's not unusual for these patients to have two or three incisions by the time the search is over. Therefore, the postoperative period is longer and more uncomfortable for these dogs than for those who have undergone a routine neuter. Anti-inflammatory drugs are often prescribed to ease the postoperative discomfort.

Home Remedies and Holistic Alternatives

Some of you may find this section interesting. Not many of us are aware of the whole world of *holistic* medicine. It is as ancient as mankind. In fact, much of what is now considered modern medicine is derived from holistic philosophy. The two have intertwining origins. A holistic approach to health incorporates a balance between mind and body, a respect for nature and natural processes, and the belief that animals as well as people fit into the scheme of nature. Both medical and spiritual forces are utilized to heal. Holistic medicine encompasses homeopathic medicine, naturopathic medicine, acupuncture, chiropractic medicine, acupressure, nutrition and herbology. Think of an holistic approach as a healthy, natural way of life. What we will do in this section is start by giving you a brief history of holistic medicine and explain how it can apply to your new puppy. Then we will give more specific examples of remedies and treatments that are purely natural.

A Brief History of Homeopathic Medicine

Words that come to mind when you hear of homeopathy might be "holistic," "natural," "botanical," "herbal," "nutritional," "naturopathic," "mind and body wholeness" and "spirituality." All these words in some ways reflect the philosophy of holistic medicine. The definition of homeopathy according to Dr. George Vithoulkas, a world-renowned homeopathic physician, is "that branch of medicine whose methodology is based on the Principles of Similars ('likes are cured by likes'). The homeopathic physician does not treat the symptoms, but considers the symptoms the outward signs of the body's attempt to cure itself."

There are three basic approaches to homeopathic medicine: nutrition, detoxification and exercise. Most people in this field consider the German physician Samuel Hahnemann the father of modern homeopathy. He was an acclaimed healer of eighteenth-century Europe who studied natural healing and the curing methods of the ancient Greeks. He once stated, "A substance that produces symptoms in a healthy person cures those symptoms in a sick person." With this in mind, he proceeded to document natural substances that caused disease-like symptoms, ultimately leading to a cure. This compilation of substances and their dosages is called the *Materia Medica*. This book has several volumes and lists alphabetically every known natural substance from botanicals to minerals, their uses in treating disease, their effects and preparations and their dosages. Remember: Many of these natural substances had been used for centuries by the ancient Romans and Greeks. Most are extracts of botanical and herbals, diluted and dissolved in water or alcohol. The concentrations may be as low as one part per million. The book ends with a *Repertory*, which is an alphabetical list of medical ailments and their homeopathic cures.

What can be said about homeopathy today? There are certainly vast differences in the medical knowledge we have versus that of over a century ago. Our understanding of medical processes has become so sophisticated as to unlock the intricate genetic codes of disease, enhance deficient immune systems, identify familial predisposition to inherited conditions and understand how viruses and cancer cells can turn a body against itself without it even putting up a fight. Even with this high level of medical comprehension, there is a whole new resurgence of homeopathy, and not just in the true believers but in people in clinical medicine, research and education. The field of homeopathy is not just a leftover from a time long gone, but an active, progressive, credible alternative to traditional Western medicine.

How Can Homeopathy Apply to Your Puppy?

The majority of veterinarians are trained in traditional medicine, just as physicians are. This is a function of the veterinary and medical colleges. There is a difference. Physicians have a choice to study traditional medicine, osteopathic medicine, naturopathic medicine or homeopathic medicine. Veterinarians only have one choice, although to be fair, veterinarians do get some homeopathic training in their curriculum.

If you're saying to yourself, "I can't imagine how or why I would ever need homeopathy," consider the following example. Let's say your veterinarian has treated your puppy for an ear infection with traditional antibiotics or antifungal medications, but with little success. Perhaps you tried another vet, then another. They all prescribed the same type of medications. In your frustration, you may consider alternative medicine. Homeopathy offers natural cures for such ailments as:

- anemia
- arthritis
- bronchitis
- colitis
- conjunctivitis
- constipation
- digestive disorders
- ear infections
- gingivitis
- kidney and urinary bladder infections

- meningitis
- muscle cramps and weakness
- nosebleeds
- sinusitis
- skin diseases
- tonsillitis and sore throats
- toothaches
- vaginitis
- vomiting and nausea

In the hands of an experienced holistic veterinarian, a whole new world of treatments and care is opened. A holistic veterinarian may treat the outer ear infection (otitis externa) by washing it with *hypericum* and *calendula* tincture, and administer botanicals such as *psorinum, mercurius corrosivus, rhus toxicodendron,* or *aconitum.* Remember, these substances may actually cause symptoms similar to otitis externa, but the philosophy is that "likes cure likes." The homeopathic vet will know how much to give (usually expressed in *centesimal* units). Dosages vary.

Examples of Homeopathic Treatments

Anemia. Anemia is a low red blood cell count. Many times this is a deficiency of iron in the diet. Foods rich in iron include green leafy vegetables, meat and liver. Instead of using medication to stimulate the bone marrow to produce more blood cells, give the body what it needs and let it produce them naturally.

Arthritis. Arthritis is an inflammation of a joint. It can be in an older dog, or in a young dog with a congenital problem (see Chapter 1 for a complete summary). The idea is to reduce the inflammation of the joint and, in so doing, reduce the pain.

In a young puppy, reduce the amount of food given; this keeps the weight down and slows the rate of growth, which can alleviate some bone growth deformities.

There are plants that have been shown to reduce joint inflammation, such as garlic, alfalfa, *rhus toxicodendron* and *ledum.*

Urinary Bladder Infection or Stones. Animals are very prone to urinary bladder infections (cystitis) and bladder stones. This is due in part to the high content of minerals in commercial diets. Other factors are 1) many animals don't naturally drink enough water to act as a natural washing mechanism; 2) many dogs are required to hold their urine until they are walked by the owner, and retention allows stagnation of the urine and encourages bacterial and yeast growth; and 3) dogs with diabetes mellitus or excessive blood sugar have excess sugar in their urine, and this sugar feeds the bacteria and yeast, allowing them to flourish. Diet is the single most important factor in preventing bladder disease. Here are a few holistic measures that can help. The emphasis is on low mineral/low sugar diets, more water intake and things that promote urination.

1. Increase water consumption to flush out the bladder and encourage sediment and sludge expulsion. This can mean adding water to the food, especially if you're feeding a dry diet, or lightly salting the food to increase water consumption.

2. Magnesium, phosphorus and calcium should be avoided. Foods rich in these minerals include dairy products, seafood and certain green leafy vegetables.

3. Avoid foods that are high in simple sugars (glucose, sucrose, dextrose and fructose). In excess, these sugars cause a rise in the blood sugar. The kidneys filter out the sugars and excrete them into the urine when they reach high levels. The sugars are food for bacteria and yeast.

4. Urinary acidifiers are helpful in lowering the pH of the urine, which in turn makes an unfavorable environment for bacteria and yeast. Such acidifiers include citrus juices, cranberry juice and vitamin C.

5. Those substances that cause diuresis (increased urine production) also aid in flushing out the urinary bladder. Natural diuretics are garlic and caffeine.

Vomiting. Puppies are very prone to nausea and vomiting. This is due to their desire to eat almost anything they can catch. It is guaranteed that if you have a puppy, it will get sick from time to time. A few holistic remedies do tend to settle an upset stomach:

1. First, withhold all food and water for twelve hours. To keep the puppy's mouth from drying out, leave out a bowl of ice cubes.

2. Second, there are foods that are bland on the stomach and easy to digest. These include white rice, boiled chicken, cottage cheese, yogurt, baby food, strained meats and crackers. These can be substituted for dog food for a couple of days while the stomach is getting back to normal.

3. Third, some natural herbs have soothing effects on an upset stomach. They are ginger, peppermint and ginseng. The mints are usually brewed into teas and drunk. Reintroduce puppy food gradually.

Pet Health Insurance

With the rising costs of high-tech veterinary services, the costs of pet health care are getting too much for many people to afford. People like the modern services that veterinarians can offer, like ultrasounds, CAT scans, bone scans, board certified specialists, intensive care units and large referral centers, just to name a few. But these high-tech procedures come with high price tags.

In human medicine, most of these procedures are covered by major medical health plans, for those fortunate enough to have health insurance. Pets are not covered under any human health plan.

Only a few underwriters in the country insure pet ailments. Their plans cover major medical expenses, but typically do not cover preventive expenses, or "well" visits or vaccines.

Several different plans are available. You should pick the one that is best for your new puppy. All plans have a deductible, which is the dollar amount you pay yourself before insurance coverage starts. Many plans have maximums per illness, which is the amount of coverage you can receive for any single illness. Then there are the annual premiums, which is the amount of money you pay to the insurance company per pet. No plan pays 100 percent of the health costs. A plan may cover only 70 percent (which means there is a 30 percent co-payment). There are the hidden catches—for example, pre-existing conditions are often excluded from coverage. Other exclusions may be birth defects, cosmetic surgery, any and all fertility/breeding and whelping costs, grooming and vaccinations.

Here are a few guidelines to use when shopping for an insurance plan (taken from the AVMA's Policy Statements and Guidelines on Pet Health Insurance and Other Third Party Animal Health Plans):

1. Pet owners should have the freedom to select a veterinarian of their choice.

2. Referrals should be allowed.

3. The policy should be accepted by the state insurance commissioner.

4. The policy should be licensed in the state in which it is sold.

Here are a few questions you should ask when shopping for a policy:

- How long has the company been insuring pet health care?
- Is the insurance carrier licensed for pet health?
- What is the annual deductible on the policy?
- What is the co-payment (the portion the insured has to pay)?
- Will it cover any pre-existing conditions?
- What is excluded from the policy—vaccines, wormings, well visits, heartworm tests, etc.?
- Are certain diseases not covered by the policy?
- What are the limits per illness, and are there annual caps?
- What is the premium payment? Is it paid all up front or monthly?
- At what age can the puppy be covered?
- Can the policy be terminated by the carrier, and for what reasons?
- Is there an upper limit to age?
- Does the puppy need to go through an exam before you can sign it up?

If your puppy is accident prone or sickly, it may be a very good idea to have it insured for accidents and illness. You may gladly pay the yearly premium instead of a stack of veterinary bills.

Chapter 5

Household Dangers and First Aid

This chapter is invaluable for anyone who fears their puppy will get into something it shouldn't. Most of us have all kinds of hidden dangers lurking in our homes. Everyday items can pose a threat to a curious puppy, who may be teething and who chews on everything in sight. Simple things like lamp cords, cleaners, antifreeze for your car, indoor plants, insects, children's toys and small items left within reach can be chewed or swallowed.

Ask any new parent, and they will tell you what they went through to child-proof their home once the child started toddling about. The same is true for puppies, except puppies toddle from the beginning. You will have to puppy-proof your home as soon as the puppy comes into it.

This chapter is divided into twelve sections:

1. Poisonous Household Plants

2. Poisonous Household Substances

3. Lamp Cord Electrocution

4. Ingestion of Foreign Objects

5. Heat Stroke

6. Choking

7. Bleeding

8. Burns

9. Bee Stings and Other Bug Bites

10. Snake Bites

11. Shock

12. CPR

Each section covers the causes, first aid treatment and prevention of each offending hazard. The chapter is full of charts that make identifying the toxin easy, as well as emergency first-aid tips you can do at home.

Poisonous Household Plants

So many of us enjoy indoor plants. They add a natural atmosphere to our homes and liven up any living space. Unfortunately, some of these household plants are toxic to pets if ingested. The effects can range from mild stomach upset to neurological problems or death. We will list the plants by their common name, followed by the symptoms associated with their toxic-

Poisonous Household Plants	
Plant Common Name	**Symptoms**
Cactus	needle injury, scratched eyes, needle in tongue
Dumb Cane	numbing of mouth, blistering in mouth, excess salivation, swollen tongue
Marijuana	hallucinations
Mistletoe†	vomiting and diarrhea, slowed pulse
Philodendron	mouth burns and blistering, throat irritation, excess salivation, swollen tongue
Poinsettia Sap	vomiting and diarrhea
Tobacco	vomiting, nausea, excess salivation, increased heart rate

† *Denotes a potentially lethal plant toxicity.*

ity. At the end, we will provide some first aid tips on removing the plant from the dog's stomach. We will also mention common toxic outdoor yard plants and ornamental garden flowers.

First Aid Considerations in Plant Poisoning

Although there are many different types of plant poisoning, a few basic first-aid techniques pertain to most. These first-aid measures in no way replace

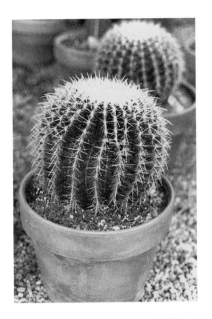
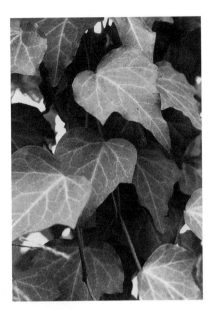
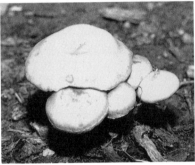

Examples of three poisonous household plants. Clockwise from upper left-hand corner: cactus, ivy and wild mushrooms.

prompt veterinary care, but these are the steps you should take immediately upon noticing the plant being eaten:

Step 1: Identify the plant. It's a good idea to know ahead of time what plants you have in your home and yard. Don't wait for an emergency to start trying frantically to identify the plant.

Step 2: Try to figure out how recently your puppy ingested the plant. Get a rough idea; was it minutes or hours ago? How much of the plant is left? Try to visualize how much of it was consumed; was it one leaf or half the plant?

Poisonous Outdoor and Garden Plants

Plant Common Name	Symptoms
Acorns[†]	kidney failure
Apple Seeds[†]	vomiting, trouble breathing, coma
Azalea Bush	excess salivation, vomiting, excess swallowing
Bird of Paradise Flower	vomiting, diarrhea, abdominal pain and cramps
Castor Bean[†]	abdominal pain, shock, low blood pressure
Cherry Tree Seeds	vomiting, trouble breathing, coma
Daffodil Flower Bulb	nausea, vomiting
English Holly	vomiting, diarrhea, abdominal pain and cramps
English Ivy Berries[†]	vomiting, diarrhea, abdominal pain and cramps
Honeysuckle	vomiting, diarrhea, abdominal pain and cramps
Horse Chestnut, nut	vomiting, diarrhea, abdominal pain and cramps
Iris Flower Bulb	vomiting, diarrhea, abdominal pain and cramps
Lily of the Valley	vomiting, diarrhea, heart arrhythmia
Morning Glory Flower	hallucinations
Nutmeg	hallucinations
Oleander[†]	vomiting, diarrhea, heart arrhythmia
Potato Skins with green buds	dry mouth, vomiting, diarrhea
Rhododendron Shrub	excess salivation, vomiting, excess swallowing
Rhubarb	vomiting, diarrhea, depression
Skunk Cabbage	burning of mouth and tongue, excess salivation, swollen throat
Tulip Bulb	vomiting, diarrhea, abdominal pain and cramps
Wild Mushroom[†]	central nervous system disturbances, coma, death
Wisteria Flower	nausea, vomiting
Yew Shrub Berries[†]	vomiting, diarrhea, wide pupils, heart arrhythmia, convulsions

[†]Denotes a potentially lethal plant toxicity.

Step 3: Call your veterinarian or local poison control center for advice. They will ask you what plant was eaten, how long ago it was eaten and how much of it was eaten. If you cannot reach anyone, go on to step 4.

Step 4: The single most important way to treat plant poisonings is to remove the source of the toxin. This usually means getting the plant out of the dog's digestive tract. There are several ways to do this.

If the plant was consumed within two hours:

1. Induce vomiting by giving either several teaspoons (for small and medium-sized dogs) or several tablespoons (for large and giant-sized dogs) of hydrogen peroxide. Repeat as needed to stimulate vomiting.

2. Another way to get a dog to vomit is by giving either one teaspoon (for small and medium-sized dogs) or one tablespoon (for large and giant-sized dogs) of the emetic Ipecac syrup. This is available in all pharmacies and is a valuable agent to stimulate vomiting. Allow the puppy to drink one cup of water, as this will hasten the vomiting. Repeat as needed.

If the plant was consumed over two hours ago:

1. Inducing vomiting will be of little help, as the plant most probably has left the stomach and is heading down the small intestine. The aim here is to move the plant material as quickly through the digestive tract as possible.

2. Use laxatives to expel the plant material quickly from the intestines. Mineral oil is safe and effective. Give one teaspoon to a small dog (under twenty-five pounds), one tablespoon to a medium-size dog (twenty-six to fifty pounds), or two tablespoons to a large or giant dog (fifty to 100 pounds). This won't work immediately, but you will see the offending plant material pass through in the stool, usually within twenty-four hours.

3. Magnesium sulfate, or Epsom salts, is another laxative you may have in the home. The dosage is $1/2$ gram per pound mixed in water, which the puppy must drink. The mixture is cathartic, so it works quicker than mineral oil and produces a very watery diarrhea.

Step 5: Call your vet! He or she can do a number of other things. A few are listed here, depending on the type of plant and the severity of the poisoning:

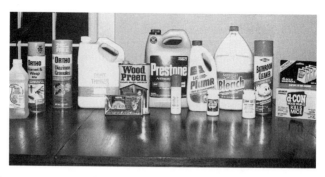

Many products we use around the home are very hazardous to puppies. Pictured here are rubbing alcohol, insect killers, antifreeze, bleach, non-aspirin pain reliever and rat killer.

- Administer IV fluids as supportive care.
- Perform gastric lavage (stomach pumping).
- Give activated charcoal to absorb the toxins.
- Give an enema to help expel the plant material from the bowel.
- Treat secondary symptoms of certain plant poisonings, like heart arrhythmia, seizure, dehydration, respiratory distress and hepatitis.

Poisonous Household Substances

This section outlines the common household, kitchen and yard substances that are toxic to puppies. Some are not going to surprise you, but others will. A general rule of thumb is that if the product label has a warning on it, then it probably is hazardous in some way. It may be a skin and eye irritant, or it may be toxic if taken internally. The one food substance that will be discussed is chocolate, which is toxic to dogs, so beware.

The following chart lists the common name of the toxic substance, the symptoms and basic first-aid steps to take while someone calls the veterinarian.

Lamp Cord Electrocution

This section deals with the puppy that finds lamp and other electric cords irresistible. Many chew on them and break through the protective plastic coating, at which time a sudden shock of electricity goes through the wet mucous membranes of the mouth. There are two forms of this I've seen. One is a mild case, with no permanent damage. The other is a serious and potentially lethal electric shock. Each is described here.

Common Household Toxic Substances

Substance	Symptoms	Basic First Aid
Acetone	vomiting diarrhea, depression, weak pulse, shock	induce vomiting[†], give baking soda in water orally
Ammonia	vomiting blood, abdominal pain, skin blisters and burns	wash skin with water and vinegar, give diluted water and vinegar orally or 3 egg whites
Antifreeze	vomiting, coma, kidney failure, death	induce vomiting[†], administer 1 oz of vodka orally followed by water, (can be repeated)
Bleach	burns of skin and mouth, vomiting	induce vomiting[†], give 3 egg whites
Carbon Monoxide	dullness, depression, dilated pupils after being in a garage with a car	mouth-to-muzzle resuscitation,* get to fresh air immediately
Charcoal Lighter	vomiting, breathing distress, shock, coma or seizures	induce vomiting[†], give laxatives[††]
Chocolate (all varieties)	vomiting, diarrhea, depression, heart arrhythmia, muscle twitching, seizures, coma from high levels of caffeine and theobromine	induce vomiting[†], give laxatives.[††] Lethal doses of 1/3 oz per lb. for dark chocolate, and 1 oz per pound for milk chocolate
Deodorants	vomiting	induce vomiting[†]
Detergents/Soap	vomiting	induce vomiting[†], give 3 egg whites or milk orally, watch breathing
Furniture Polish	vomiting, breathing distress, shock, coma or seizures	induce vomiting[†], give laxatives[††]
Gasoline	skin irritation, weakness, dementia, dilated pupils, vomiting, twitching	induce vomiting[†], give vegetable oil orally to block absorption, get into fresh air
Ibuprofin (Advil™)	vomiting, stomach ulceration, kidney failure	induce vomiting[†], give laxatives[††] many need IV fluids
Kerosene/Fuel Oil	vomiting, breathing distress, shock, coma or seizures	induce vomiting[†], give laxatives,[††] give vegetable oil orally to block absorption

Mouth-to-muzzle resuscitation is described later in this chapter.

Substance	Symptoms	Basic First Aid
Lead	vomiting, diarrhea, anemia, neurologic symptoms, blindness, seizures, coma	induce vomiting[†], give laxatives, remove source of lead (paint chips, car battery, leaded gasoline, plumbing solder, grease, pellets, fishing anchors, golf balls, shotgun shot)
Lime	skin irritant, burns	wash skin with copious soap and water
Lye	vomiting blood, abdominal pain, skin blisters and burns	wash skin with water and vinegar, give diluted water and vinegar orally or 3 egg whites
Organophosphate Insecticides	excess drooling, weakness, seizures, vomiting, dilated pupils	wash off insecticide, administer atropine sulfate as the antidote
Paint Thinner	vomiting, breathing distress, shock, coma or seizures	induce vomiting[†], give laxatives[††]
Phenol Cleaners	nausea, vomiting, shock, liver or kidney failure	wash off skin, induce vomiting[†], give 3 egg whites or milk orally
Rat Poison	excess bleeding, anemia, cyanosis	induce vomiting[†], requires vitamin K injections
Rubbing Alcohol	weakness, incoordination, blindness, coma, dilated pupils, vomiting and diarrhea	induce vomiting[†], give baking soda in water to neutralize acidosis
Strychnine	dilated pupils, respiratory distress, rigid muscles, seizures and spasms with loud noises or stimulus, brown urine	induce vomiting[†], keep dog in a dark quiet room until taking him to the veterinarian
Turpentine	vomiting, diarrhea, bloody urine, neurologic disorientation, coma, breathing distress	induce vomiting[†], give vegetable oil by mouth to block absorption, give laxatives[††]
Tylenol™	depression, fast heart rate, brown urine, anemia	induce vomiting[†], give 500 mg vitamin C per 25 lb., followed by baking soda in water

[†]***Induce vomiting*** *by giving several teaspoons (for small and medium-size dogs), or several tablespoons (for large and giant-size dogs) of hydrogen peroxide orally. Repeat as needed to stimulate vomiting. Another remedy 1 teaspoon (for small and medium dogs) or 1 tablespoon (for large and giant dogs) of Ipecac syrup. Allow the puppy to drink 1 cup of water, as this will hasten the vomiting. Repeat as needed.*

[††] ***Laxatives*** *are used to quickly expel the plant material from the intestines. Mineral oil is safe and effective. Give 1 teaspoon for small dogs (under 25 lb.), 1 tablespoon to a medium-size dog (26-50 lb.), and 2 tablespoons to a large or giant dog (50-100 lb.).*

Mild Shock from an Electric Cord

We've all had a shock from a wall outlet sometime in our lives. Most of us walk away from it with little more than a tingling sensation in our finger. It doesn't hurt as much as it startles and scares us. For a small puppy, the shock can be more than that.

In the instant the shock occurs, the electric current flows through the mouth mucous membranes, often leaving burns. On inspection, you can actually see the black marks where the burn occurred, surrounded by swollen red, blistered tissue. The puppy may seem dazed for several minutes immediately following the shock. There will be excess salivation, and the puppy

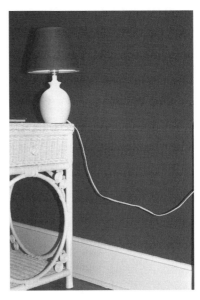

This lamp and its exposed cord are a perfect target for a playful pup, which could be electrocuted chewing on the cord.

often runs around the room crying, trying to run away from the pain.

The treatment is twofold. First, you should try to reduce the pain and swelling in the mouth by applying ice cubes to the burn, which will numb the area and keep the swelling down. Second, if there are second- or third-degree burns, you can apply antibiotic oral gel to the burns to keep them from becoming infected. Luckily, the mouth of a dog is naturally clean. The puppy may not eat solid or dry food for several days because it hurts. We all know how painful a small canker sore can be. Just imagine a third-degree burn!

The mouth heals quickly, and little follow-up attention is required. Contact your vet to see whether something else needs to be done.

Severe Shock from an Electric Cord

A young, small-breed puppy could actually be electrocuted from an electric cord. The amperage of a typical house is anywhere from fifteen to thirty amperes per circuit, carrying 120 volts. This is enough to kill a small dog. With any luck the puppy will live, but immediate life-saving steps are needed.

The biologic changes during an electrocution are the following:

1. Second- and third-degree burns to the mouth

2. Heart arrhythmia

3. Acute pulmonary (lung) fluid infiltration

These dogs show symptoms of unconsciousness, blackened mouth and gums, breathing distress, circulatory shock and possible seizure. You can do very little at home to treat this. These puppies need immediate professional help. The only thing you can do at home is start CPR and mouth-to-muzzle resuscitation, as described later in this chapter. Veterinarians treat electrocution aggressively with oxygen therapy and respirators, anti-arrhythmia heart drugs, supportive IV fluid therapy for shock, diuretics to remove the fluid accumulation in the lungs and antibiotics for preventing pneumonia. The prognosis is *guarded*.

Ingestion of Foreign Objects

Puppies are notorious for eating small objects off the floor and countertops. As part of puppy-proofing your home, remove all objects that could fit in the palm of your hand from floors, chairs, counters and closets. Wastebaskets in bathrooms and kitchens are another source of objects. The point here is that these puppies are constantly scouring the floors looking for things to chew on, and eventually swallow.

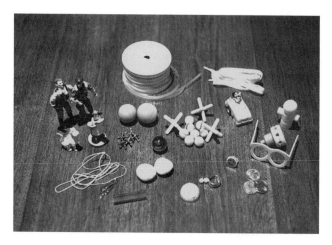

Some of the objects puppies might swallow by accident are toy figurines, string, jacks, marbles, coins, shoelaces, and paper clips.

You can't believe the things a dog will eat. Here is just a partial list of things I have seen:

bones	gloves	rocks
children's toys	handballs	rubber bands
Christmas ornaments	marbles	sanitary tampons
coins	panty hose	shoelaces
cooking knives	paper clips	socks
crayons	pens or pencils	sponges
earrings	plastic bags	tennis balls
electric cord plugs	ribbon	toilet paper
fish hooks	rings	rocks

Each veterinarian could add his or her own findings to this list. The point is that many things in our everyday life are potential hazards to a puppy. Also, certain breeds are more prone to eating foreign objects due to their mouthing instinct. Most sporting breeds fit this description. Perhaps the Retriever is the most notorious. Just be aware of this problem.

Symptoms are basically the same regardless of the object swallowed. The puppy starts vomiting, gagging, dry heaving and coughing. This may persist for hours, or intermittently for days. The puppy stops eating and drinking, or if it tries to eat or drink, the food or water comes right up. After a day or so of this, most owners become concerned. At this point, the puppy may be obstructed, meaning that the object has blocked the natural flow of materials through the intestine. Intestinal obstructions are life-threatening.

Upon presentation at the veterinary office, the puppy is weak, hunched over, suffering pain in the abdomen and has pale mucous membranes. The dog may be salivating from the nausea. If the object is large enough, the vet may be able to palpate it in the abdomen.

Since these symptoms are nonspecific and can be from numerous other problems, including poisonings, viral enteritis, pancreatitis, gallstone attack, gastric or duodenal ulcer, acute kidney failure, food poisoning and bloat, it is very important to get a firm diagnosis of foreign body gastroenteritis. The diagnosis is made in one of several ways, in order of progression:

1. Physical exam

2. Plain radiology (X rays without any contrast media)

3. Contrast radiology (such as an upper GI series with barium)

4. Ultrasonography (abdominal ultrasound imaging)

5. Endoscopy (a flexible fiberoptic tube with a lens passed into the stomach to visualize objects)

6. Exploratory surgery (the final frontier; examination of stomach and intestines)

The veterinarian may not need to do all of the preceding. A diagnosis may be made after only the first or second test. Once the diagnosis is made and the object is identified, the next step is to try to get the material to pass out of the body. In some cases, the veterinary surgeon will need to remove the object surgically. I have often tried large doses of mineral oil with great success. If the patient isn't too debilitated, dehydrated or uncomfortable, the mineral oil can be given. A large quantity may be four to six tablespoons orally for a seventy-five-pound Labrador. This dose can be repeated twice, eight to twelve hours apart. Since mineral oil is an intestinal laxative, it must get to where the object is in order to work. It takes a minimum of twelve to twenty-four hours for this to happen. If the object isn't too large, it will start to pass in this time. The key is knowing when to say, "We've waited a good twenty-four hours. Nothing passed. It's time to consider surgery before the dog becomes more debilitated or the intestine ruptures."

Once the object is out of the body, the dog seems to respond almost immediately. If surgery was performed, there is a recuperative period of several days during which only liquefied foods are given. If the mineral oil passed the object, the dog can resume normal eating.

The key to successful treatment of foreign body ingestion is to get an early, accurate diagnosis and prompt treatment.

Heat Stroke

Heat stroke is also known as *hyperthermia*. This is when the body core temperature exceeds 105°F. Breeds most prone to this are those with a reduced passage of air through their nostrils, such as the breeds with pushed-in faces (Pekingese, Bulldog, Lhasa Apso, Boston Terrier and Pug). The only place on a dog's body where it can sweat is the pads of its feet; therefore, a dog relies on panting to cool the body. Anything that restricts the air flow through the nasal passages of a dog will increase its chances of overheating. The most notorious cause of heat stroke in dogs is enclosure in a hot car on a warm day with closed windows. These dogs can become overheated in under thirty minutes.

The symptoms of impending heat stroke are intense panting, very ruddy mucous membranes, weakness, racing heart rate, fainting, excess salivation, coma and, eventually, death. If the dog remains hyperthermic for more than ten minutes, irreparable brain damage may occur due to brain swelling.

There isn't much time to waste in these cases. Whether the dog survives depends on removing the dog from the dangerous environment and cooling the body off gradually. Try to lower the body temperature by bathing in cool (not ice-cold) water. We look for a 1°F drop every five minutes. Get the puppy to a veterinarian quickly so that other supportive measures can be instituted. Only time will tell whether there was permanent brain or organ system damage. *Please, never leave your dog in a closed car on a warm day (anything over 68°F)! The air cannot circulate in a closed car, and it becomes as hot as a sauna. This quickly becomes life-threatening for a dog.*

Choking

Choking is a frightening thing. Puppies are particularly susceptible to it because they are always chewing on something. No matter how many times you pull something out of their mouths, there will be a time when you will miss something. When a puppy is chewing on an object and then takes a deep breath (to bark or pant, or when startled), the object can become lodged in the back of the throat. This obstructs air flow and is considered choking. Immediately, the puppy starts to cough, gasp or heave. You may think the puppy is trying to vomit, but it quickly becomes apparent that its air is shut off. Within thirty to sixty seconds, the puppy becomes cyanotic (blue from lack of oxygen) and may pass out. There are four techniques you can use to treat choking.

1. The first is to try to pull out the object with your fingers. The problems with this are that the puppy is struggling, there is the chance you may be bitten, and the suction created from the dog gasping makes it difficult to pull it out.

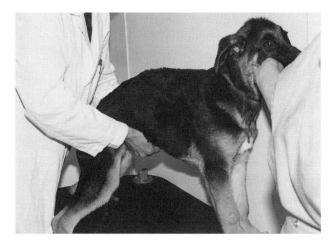

A choking dog may need the Heimlich maneuver to help expel a stuck object. It's performed by grasping both fists together and forcibly pushing them into the dog's diaphragm.

2. The second method is a variation of the *Heimlich maneuver*. With this technique, you grasp your fists together and forcibly push them into the dog's abdomen just behind the sternum. Your thrusting motion pushes on the diaphragm, which in turn forces air out the windpipe. This often dislodges the object. Do this vigorously, and repeat several times. If the puppy is unconscious, you can maneuver better, so keep trying.

3. The third method of treating choking involves performing a tracheotomy, or making a hole in the windpipe. This is typically done by a veterinarian.

Bleeding

Cuts and scrapes are a part of every puppy's life. The superficial ones are of no concern and usually heal with little or no treatment. This section deals with bleeding of a more serious nature (an exception is bleeding from nails, which is discussed in Chapter 4). Another word for this is *hemorrhage*, or profuse bleeding that should be stopped, or else anemia and other profound changes can occur that are life-threatening. There are three types of hemorrhage: venous, arterial and capillary.

1. The *venous* form is from a vein. Veins are the blood vessels that carry used (deoxygenated) blood from the body back to the heart and lungs. They are under a steady pressure, much lower than that of arteries. When a vein is punctured or cut, a steady drip, ooze or stream of blood flows from it. Think of it as a cut in a garden hose that is under low constant pressure. An example of a venous hemorrhage is a cut pad from stepping on glass.

2. The second form is *arterial* hemorrhage. This is when an artery is severed. Arteries are the blood vessels that carry the oxygen-rich blood through the body. They are under higher pressure than veins, and the pressure isn't constant but pulsates with every heartbeat. The blood spurts out of a cut artery in a rhythmic pattern. The blood loss is usually much faster in arterial hemorrhages due to the higher pressure. This form of hemorrhage is the most serious. An example of an arterial hemorrhage is a deep cut in between the toes, severing a toe artery.

3. The third form is *capillary* bleeding, which is common whenever there is trauma to areas that have capillary beds, such as the eyes, ears, or mucous membranes of nose, mouth and skin. Capillary beds ooze blood. You don't see the spurting you see in arterial hemorrhages. Examples of capillary bleeding are nosebleeds and skin bruises.

Regardless of the type of hemorrhage, it must be stopped at once. We will go over the basics of first aid for hemorrhage control. The techniques for each type of hemorrhage are outlined here.

To Stop Venous Bleeding:

1. Raise the affected body part above the level of the heart.

2. Apply pressure sufficient to stop or at least slow down the bleeding.

3. Try to wrap the area with bandaging, cloth strips, a towel, a shredded T-shirt, an Ace bandage or anything else you may have. Apply it tightly enough so that it won't fall off, but not so tightly as to stop all circulation.

4. Apply ice packs to the area. Cold temperatures slow down blood flow.

To Stop Arterial Bleeding, do steps 1–3, above, then:

4. In cases of spurting blood that a bandage cannot stop (the blood keeps soaking through the bandage), a tourniquet needs to be applied. A tourniquet is a strap that gets applied above the wound, shutting off the blood supply to that area. Since most of these deep lacerations are on the paw, the tourniquet placement is on the leg, above the wrist (for a front leg) or hock (for a hind leg). A *tourniquet* can be made from string, strips of cloth, a belt, a rubber band or anything that can be tied around a limb. It has to be tight enough to stop the circulation, which means that below it the area will be cold and purple-colored. *A tourniquet can stay on for only ten to fifteen minutes before permanent damage to the limb occurs. If it takes longer than that to get to a veterinary facility, you have to release the tourniquet every ten to fifteen minutes for three to five minutes to allow blood flow.* During that time, you will have to use your hands and a cloth to apply pressure directly to the cut to keep the bleeding under control.

To Stop Capillary Bleeding:

1. Apply pressure sufficient to stop or at least slow down the bleeding.

2. If the bleeding is from a scrape and a large area of skin is bleeding, use a soft cloth to apply gentle pressure on top of the wound. Wrap cloth or bandaging material around the area to keep a constant, low pressure on the wound. The goal is just to cover the wound. These wounds just ooze blood and don't bleed profusely like the high-pressure venous or arterial wounds.

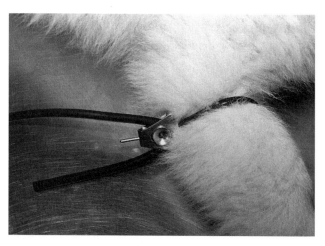

This is a professional veterinary tourniquet to stop bleeding. You can make your own with a cloth strap.

3. Apply ice packs to the area; cold temperatures slow down blood flow.

4. In the event of a nosebleed, try to use a tissue to apply pressure inside the nostril. Always keep the nose elevated. Use ice packs on the side of the muzzle. If you have a nasal decongestant spray in the house, you can give one spray in the bleeding nostril. This constricts the capillaries and slows down the bleeding. Always have nosebleeds checked by your veterinarian, as they can be a symptom of another ailment.

Burns

Burns can be caused by three different sources: thermal, chemical and electrical. Regardless of the type, all of them hurt a great deal and cause tissue destruction. The skin is usually the tissue that gets burned. There are three different types of skin burns:

First Degree. These burns are superficial. The top layer of skin, called the epidermis, is involved. The area becomes red and very painful, and the top layer of skin is usually lost.

Second Degree. These burns are deeper, involving the epidermis and part of the deeper dermal layers of the skin. These burns are very painful and bleed or ooze. They take longer to heal and are more serious than the superficial burns. Blistering is common.

Third Degree. These burns are the most severe and involve the full thickness of the skin. The epidermis and dermis are destroyed. The skin appears to melt away, exposing the deeper tissues underneath. The area becomes red, swollen and blackened; bleeding may be minimal because the blood vessels are also destroyed. These burns can be life-threatening if 50 percent or more of the body surface is involved. These animals will be in shock and require immediate medical care.

Possible sources of the three different types of burns are listed here. You may be surprised to find how many different common household things can cause burns.

Thermal Burn Sources:

candles	hot water pipes and risers
car mufflers and tailpipes	hot plates
fireplaces	ovens
flames	radiators
furnaces	scalding water
heating pads	stoves

Chemical Burn Sources:

acetone	kerosene
ammonia	lime
asphalt	liquid drain cleaners
bathroom cleaners	lye
battery acid	paint thinner
bleach	phenol cleaners
flooring adhesive	road salt
gasoline	

Electrical Burn Sources:

car batteries	hobby batteries
electrical cords	lamp cords
extension cords	wall outlets

First Aid for Burns

1. Remove the source of the burn.

2. If chemical, flush area with lots of water.

3. Run the affected area under cold water, or apply ice packs.

4. If superficial, apply topical antibiotic ointment twice daily.

5. If deeper or full thickness, seek veterinary care.

6. Cover with a light bandage to keep clean.

Bee Stings and Other Bug Bites

Most insect bites are an annoyance and cause itching and swelling at the bite site. Some, however, are more serious. If your puppy is allergic to bee stings, its reaction can be serious. Dogs can be as allergic to bee stings as some people. The bites and stings of the following insects have been known to cause severe reactions in puppies:

- fire ants
- brown spiders
- black widow spiders
- wasps
- honeybees
- bumblebees
- hornets
- yellowjackets

At the very least, the bug bite usually causes a local reaction of swelling, pain, ulceration and redness of the skin, which can last for days. The dog scratches at it and can make an infected mess of it. Treating with topical cortisone and antibiotic ointments can prevent this. If the bite is venomous, there are systemic reactions as well. These might include fever, joint pain, muscle aching, vomiting and diarrhea, and a generalized allergic reaction called *Anaphylaxis*.

Anaphylaxis is a sudden, intense, allergic reaction that causes respiratory failure and can be fatal within minutes. Once an allergic substance enters the body, *histamine* is released from certain cells in the immune system. If a small amount of histamine is released, there will be only a local reaction: hives, redness, swelling and itching. If, however, a massive amount of histamine is released, the entire body goes into *histamine shock*, in which blood pressure drops and the lungs fill up with fluid within minutes. The animal quickly goes into shock and respiratory and cardiac failure, and dies.

The only way to stop this violent reaction is to administer the antidote to histamine, namely *adrenaline* (also called *epinephrine*). Bee-sting kits are available that inject a preset dose of epinephrine to counteract the histamine. I recommend that if you have a dog with a known hypersensitivity to bee stings, you may want your veterinarian to prescribe one of these in case of emergency. Make sure you have the right size of antidote for your dog (the antidotes come in different sizes) and that you know how to use it. The time to learn how to use it is not when you need it. Getting your puppy to a veterinarian is of critical importance. Timing in these cases is everything. Your veterinarian will treat the shock and fluid accumulation in the lungs, reverse the histamine reaction, and keep the puppy for observation.

Snake Bites

There are many different snakes in this country, and the vast majority of them are nonvenomous: Although these snakes can bite, they don't carry any poison; but they can still leave nasty bites that can become infected. The fear involved in any snake bite situation is not knowing whether the snake was poisonous. There are ways to tell them apart, and you should learn what they are to prepare yourself.

The poisonous snakes in North America are pit vipers. These snakes have a hole (pit) between their eye and nostril, they have elliptical pupils instead of round ones like the harmless snakes, and they have large fangs. The pit vipers found in North America are

- cobras
- copperheads
- coral snakes
- cottonmouths
- diamondback rattlesnakes
- rattlesnakes
- water moccasins

The symptoms of a snake bite are explosive swelling around the two fang holes, bruising and disfigurement of the face (if the bite was there). Neurological symptoms, with seizures, coma and death, can ensue within two to four hours. The timing of the treatment is critical. The last snake bite I treated was on a ninety-pound black Labrador named Jake who was bitten on the upper lip by a cottonmouth. The face was so swollen that the eyes were shut, and he was having trouble breathing. Neurological symptoms hadn't started yet because the owner was able to bring him to me within thirty minutes. The two fang holes were bleeding. Jake survived the bite, but not without weeks of recovery. I had to treat him aggressively with IV fluids, opening and flushing the bite holes and injections of antivenin (the antidote I got from the local human hospital).

First Aid for Snake Bites

There are steps that you can take to increase the chances of your puppy's survival in the event of a snake bite:

1. Do not stress the dog or make it move unnecessarily. This only spreads the venom faster. Keep the dog lying flat.

2. Tie a string, belt, strip of cloth or anything else you may have that can act like a tourniquet above the bite if it is on a limb. This slows down venous circulation and impedes the spread of the venom. Loosen the tourniquet every ten to fifteen minutes so as not to obstruct blood flow completely.

3. Try to flush out bite holes with water or hydrogen peroxide. The old *Boy Scouts of America Handbook* used to recommend sucking out the wounds by mouth if a fellow scout was bitten. Use your own discretion. They now have kits with a suction.

4. Get your puppy to a veterinary facility as fast as you can. Some venom only takes a couple of hours to kill an animal.

The veterinarian will immediately start intravenous fluids, treatment for shock and antivenin injections to neutralize the venom. Even with all this timely treatment, the prognosis is *guarded.*

Shock

Shock is a term we use to describe when there is dangerously low blood pressure or blood circulation to the crucial areas of the body (brain, muscles or major organ systems). There are several different types of shock:

1. Shock due to sudden blood loss

2. Shock due to sudden drop in blood pressure

3. Shock due to fright and trauma

Shock is a life-threatening condition. The danger is that not enough blood reaches the critical areas of the body, which can lead to irreparable damage to nerve tissue, brain, kidney, cardiac muscle, and major organ systems. The body makes an attempt to increase the blood flow to these crucial areas while shutting off blood flow to not-so-critical ones, like the intestines. Life cannot be sustained for long if crucial organs are not functioning. If permanent damage occurs, the animal will die. This is why it is so important to try to reverse these changes during shock as quickly as possible.

The symptoms for shock are the same regardless of the type or cause. The most noticeable are these:

- Low blood pressure
- Increased heart rate to try to compensate for low blood pressure
- Quick breathing as an attempt to increase the oxygenation of the blood
- Unconsciousness or disorientation
- Fixed dilated pupils
- Collapse, fainting·or coma

A veterinarian will treat shock very aggressively with intravenous fluids, drugs to increase the blood pressure and blood perfusion of the organs. If bleeding is the cause, it must be stopped first. A blood transfusion may be needed if there has been a 30 percent loss of blood. Some common methods and drugs used to treat shock are outlined in the following table. Some of these you can do; others must be done by a veterinarian.

If the following steps are taken, the chances are best for your puppy to survive the shock. Signs that your efforts are working are the following:

- Breathing becomes regular and slower.
- The color of the mucous membranes becomes pink again.
- The heart rate slows down to normal (between seventy and 150 beats per minute), and the pulses feel full and strong.
- The urinary bladder starts to fill again.
- Body temperature rises to normal (between 100-101°F).
- Consciousness returns.

CPR

There are times when a dog goes into cardiac arrest and needs to be resuscitated. Cardiac arrest is when the heart stops beating or beats in an abnormal way, causing a sudden drop in blood pressure. Events that may bring on acute cardiac arrest are

- acute viral and bacterial diseases
- electrocution
- getting hit by lightning
- poisonings (see pages 168–172)
- shock (see above)
- trauma (like being hit by a car)

Shock Therapy	
Treatment or Procedure	Effect on System
IV fluids†	Increase blood volume to improve perfusion of organ systems
Open airway	This ensures that there is no obstruction to breathing
Stop all bleeding	Hemorrhage control measures for arterial and venous hemorrhage
Keep in lying position	This keeps the blood flow directed to the head and brain where it is most crucial
Keep warm with heating pads and blankets	During shock, body temperature usually falls, causing hypothermia (to temperatures below 99°F)
Blood transfusions†	This corrects blood loss of more than 30%
Check for heart rate beats and quality of pulse	Heart rate usually increases during shock (150–250 beats per minute), and the pulses get weak and "thready"
Check mucus membrane color and capillary refill time	The mucus membranes of the mouth become white in shock, and when you press on the gums, it takes more than 2 seconds for the color to come back
Monitor for urine output, if none, increase IV fluids and give Diuretic drugs†	When the blood perfusion to the kidneys is low, urine production will stop; this is reversed by increasing the amount of fluids given intravenously, and with diuretic drugs that increase urine production
Injections of Cortisone†	This drug stabilizes blood vessels, increases oxygenation of the blood, and increases blood flow

†Denotes must be performed by a veterinarian.

There are three main objectives to CPR. They are the **ABC**s of **CPR**:

A is for *airway.* You must establish a patent airway.

B is for *breathing.* You must breathe for the animal.

C is for *cardiac* **function.** You must help pump the blood from the heart.

Let's go through each one. The key to successful CPR is timing. Starting immediately and performing the procedure correctly are the keys to success. Never be afraid to start CPR. If the animal responds quickly, you can stop. All you've wasted was some time and effort.

A is for Airway:

The first thing you must do when a dog goes down, unconscious and in shock, is to keep an open breathing airway. Make sure that nothing is caught in the throat and that the dog isn't swallowing its tongue. Position the head so that it is outstretched and not bent. Pull out the tongue so that it is not in the back of the throat. Remove any foam or froth that might be in the back of the throat, using a paper towel.

B is for Breathing:

Since the dog isn't breathing, you must breathe for it. This is done with a procedure we call "mouth-to-muzzle" resuscitation.

1. If the puppy (a Pekingese, for example) has a short muzzle, put your mouth over the entire face of the dog so that its nose and mouth are in your mouth. Blow air into the dog by exhaling. Don't do this with all your force. Do it enough to make the chest inflate slightly; then release the pressure by taking your mouth away. Do this every twenty-five to thirty seconds.

2. If the breed has a long muzzle and snout, you can cup your hands together to form a tunnel. Keep the dog's mouth closed, and wrap your cupped hands around the dog's nose. Blow air by exhaling into your hand-tunnel until you see the dog's chest inflate slightly. Then release the pressure by taking your hands away from the nose. Do this every twenty-five to thirty seconds.

C is for Cardiac:

Since most dogs in this condition are in acute heart failure, their heart isn't beating or pumping blood efficiently, if at all. You must help pump the blood for the dog. Do this by laying the dog on its side and clasping your hands together, on top of the other. You need to kneel down beside the dog, bend over its chest, and place your left hand over the heart area of the chest. Then place your right hand on top of your left one, perpendicular to it. Lean over and, with your weight, push down in short bursts of pressure over the heart. This is pumping action. Push on the chest, count to five, and then do it again. Keep repeating this procedure for five to ten minutes or until you can get to a veterinary facility.

It is preferable for two people to be performing CPR at the same time. One person does the heart pumping; the other, the breathing. If you are alone, you must alternate between breathing and pumping as best you can.

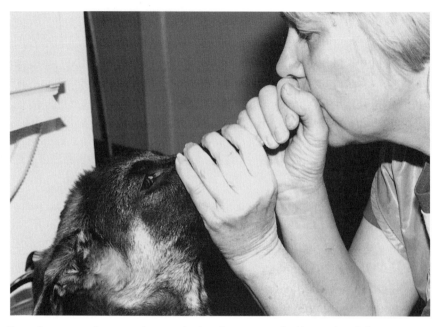

To perform mounth-to-muzzle resuscitation, form a tunnel with your hands between your mouth and the dog's muzzle.

During the CPR process, you should be checking for signs that the dog is responding. If you see any of these, celebrate! You may have saved your puppy's life. These signs are the following:

- Breathing starts on its own.
- A pink color returns to the mucous membranes of the mouth.
- A strong heartbeat can be felt through the chest (between the third and fifth ribs).
- Consciousness returns.
- Pupils return to normal size.

Chapter 6

Puppy Pediatrics

This chapter is perhaps the most useful of all. It covers in detail all the common diseases of puppies. Collectively, we call this focus *pediatrics,* meaning the study of childhood diseases. This chapter is designed to be a reference guide for most common medical disorders of young dogs. If your veterinarian diagnoses a problem, you can use this chapter to look up the disease and educate yourself about it. Maybe you'll have questions for your vet after reading the section on the disease. The chapter is organized into eight sections:

1. Skin and Coat Diseases

2. Eye, Ear and Throat Diseases

3. Respiratory Diseases

4. Gastrointestinal Diseases

5. Hormonal Diseases

6. Musculoskeletal Diseases

7. Neurological Diseases

8. Urogenital Diseases

Each section covers the most common puppy problems in that group, including the disease process, symptoms, diagnosis, treatment, and prognosis (where appropriate). *We will not reiterate diseases of a congenital or inherited nature or those described in detail in other chapters.*

Skin and Coat Diseases

Skin diseases constitute a large portion of pediatric problems. We will cover the most common skin disorders of puppies under one year of age. Some are inconsequential; others are serious. Infectious, environmental, cancerous and allergic conditions are covered.

Impetigo and the "Staph" Connection

Perhaps the most common skin disease of young puppies under six months of age is impetigo, a *Staphylococcus intermedius* infection of the skin. This bacterium is notorious in skin infections in children and almost all species of animals. It is considered opportunistic, meaning it just waits for an abrasion through which it can enter the skin. Infection can involve the hair follicles or bald areas and causes small whiteheads. Another word for infections of the hair follicles is *folliculitis*. This can happen just from the puppy scratching at its skin or from the mother licking the puppy. The most common site is in between the hind legs, in the groin area, in the armpits and on the inner thighs, where the skin gets soiled with urine and feces. Most of these infections are superficial, meaning only involving the upper layers of the skin; however, if left untreated, they can progress to deep infections called deep pyoderma, furunculosis or puppy strangles (see "Puppy Strangles").

The skin becomes swollen and red, with pus exuding from open sores. There are often whiteheads and itching, and the puppy is irritated in that area. Diagnosis is made by clinical observation of the patient, as well as a bacterial culture of the discharge that oozes out of the pimples. Make sure a sensitivity is also done as part of the culture, as *Staphylococcus* bacteria are resistant to many common antibiotics. *Staphylococcus* bacteria can make an enzyme, called β-lactamase, which blocks the effects of many antibiotics.

Bacterial skin infections are treated with frequent washings of the skin, warm compresses to enhance healing, topical antibiotic ointments and oral antibiotics if the infection is spreading or appears deeper than superficial. Impetigo is usually a direct result of poor hygiene, so attempts to wash the puppy's skin with an antibacterial soap daily will greatly reduce the disease. As mentioned previously, make sure the veterinarian chooses an antibiotic that is proven to kill the specific strain on the sensitivity report. Most puppies eventually become immune to *Staphylococcus* bacteria. Therefore, it's a common disease of puppies under six months old. The prognosis is *good*.

Hot Spots and Pyoderma

The *Staphylococcus* infection described in the "Impetigo" section describes superficial skin infections. "Hot spots" and deep pyoderma are skin infections involving the deeper layers of the skin. They often start as an itch or irritation, such as an insect bite. A local hive or wheal develops, and the dog

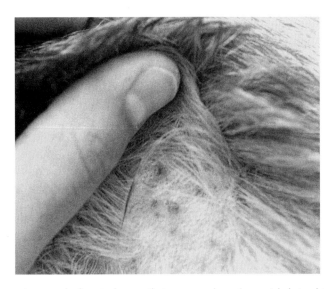

Hot spots are large, red, ulcerated areas that are anywhere from nickel-sized to six inches in diameter.

itches and scratches. As mentioned in the preceding section, *Staphylococcus* bacteria are opportunistic, meaning they invade the skin once it has a break. As the dog continues to itch, more and more of the skin layers become involved, until the infection is deep within the dermis. Instead of whiteheads and pimples apearing (as is the case in impetigo), large, red, ulcerated areas form that bleed and are very painful. There may even be a bull's-eye in the center where the infection started. These areas can be anywhere from nickel-sized to six inches in diameter.

Because this can look like other skin ailments of dogs, a firm diagnosis is important to rule out fungal infection, fleas, mange and autoimmune diseases. The veterinarian may take cultures and skin scrapings, and shave the hair immediately around the infection so as to make it easier to keep it clean.

Treatment usually includes prescribing antibiotics and/or topical anti-inflammatory drugs. It's important to keep the dog from scratching or licking at the infection, or it won't heal. If it can be bandaged, then do so. If not, then an Elizabethan neck collar will keep the dog from getting to the hot spot. The essentials to treating a hot spot are threefold: 1) antibiotics for the infection, 2) anti-inflammatory drugs and anti-itch to calm the itch and reduce the pain and swelling, and 3) a bandage or covering to keep the puppy from making the infection worse. If the hot spot is on the trunk of the body, putting a T-shirt on the puppy so that it covers that area will keep the puppy from licking. It may take a few weeks for a severe case to heal. With proper care, these infections usually heal, carrying a *good* prognosis.

Puppy Strangles

This is the third form of *Staphylococcus* infection in young puppies. It is more of a localized explosive infection that occurs when there is a hypersensitivity (allergy) to the bacteria. Areas usually affected are the face and neck. The swelling can get so extreme that the eyes swell shut and the neck lymph nodes get large enough to make breathing difficult. There is often a discharge that breaks from the swelling, draining blood and pus. Since the puppy is allergic to the bacteria, much of the swelling is due to that, as opposed to infection.

Treatment should be instituted right away. Warm compresses enhance healing and drainage of the pus. Antibiotics are used to treat the infection. Cortisone drugs are given to counteract the hypersensitivity and reduce swelling. All three must be done for this disease to be cured. There is often some scarring and disfigurement of the areas with the worst swelling and draining tracts. It often takes five to ten days to see an initial improvement. The prognosis is *guarded* during the initial phase of the disease and *fair* once the swelling subsides.

Allergic Dermatitis (Atopy)

Dogs have allergies and allergic reactions just like people do. If the dog comes into contact with something it's allergic to (called an allergen), which comes into contact with the skin or is breathed in, a chain of events leads to an allergic reaction. What exactly is an allergy? An *allergy* is a bodily reaction against a substance to which the individual has a sensitivity. In other words, if your dog is allergic to dust and goes into the back of a closet that hasn't been dusted in years, the dust will get into your dog's eyes, nose and respiratory system. Once there, the body reacts to it by causing inflammation, swelling and pain locally. There are also secretions along with the inflammation. In the eye, the secretions are in the form of excessive tearing; in the nose, it will be a clear, watery discharge; and in the sinuses and lungs, it will be thicker mucus. The skin reacts by becoming inflamed, red and itchy, and may break out in hives. The hair may eventually fall out.

What causes this allergic reaction? To continue with the dust example, once the dust makes contact with cells lining the eyelids, nose, sinus or bronchi, the dust combines with antibodies matched to it. What determines whether your dog will have antibodies to dust? Two things: 1) previous and

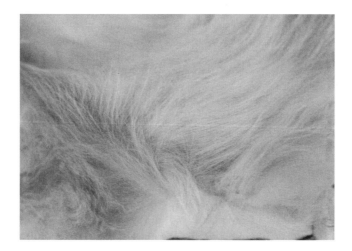

An allergic skin reaction manifests itself as an inflamed, red, itchy area.

prolonged exposure to dust, and 2) genetics. This union between allergen and antibody then stimulates various cells of the immune system to release chemical mediators of the allergic reaction. These chemical mediators start the allergic process in the body.

Most allergies that affect the skin of puppies are *delayed*. What this means is that those dogs allergic to things don't show symptoms immediately but have to develop a sensitivity over time. What kinds of things can cause an allergic reaction in a dog's skin?

- Aerosol sprays
- Bird feathers
- Bug bites (spider, ant and bee)
- Carpet cleaners
- Carpet fibers
- Carpet matting
- Certain foods
- Cosmetics
- Dust
- Flea bites
- Fumes from construction products
- Grass, tree and other plant pollens
- Mold spores
- Other animal dander
- Smoke
- Upholstery stuffing
- Wool fibers

You can see that all of us have some of these in our houses. If your puppy is developing a chronic allergy that is causing skin rash, itching, hives and hair loss, you may want to try to find out what your dog is allergic to. There are two ways your veterinarian can do this.

Skin Testing. This is where your veterinarian injects minute amounts of dozens of different allergens along with histamine (as the control) into the dermis layer of your puppy's skin (called an *intradermal* injection). The vet waits a specified period of time, then measures the diameter of the hive that develops if an allergic reaction has occurred. It is considered a positive reaction if the hive is equal to or greater in diameter than the hive produced by the histamine injection. As you can imagine, this is time-consuming, tedious and uncomfortable for your puppy. For these reasons, this method is considered a bit antiquated.

RAST (Radioallergosorbent Test). This is the test of choice for most veterinarians these days. It is done with a blood sample from the patient, without all those intradermal injections. The test detects the presence of the specific antibodies to their allergens. In other words, if your puppy is allergic to dust, there will be a high level of dust-antibodies in its blood. Most RAST tests will tests for dozens of outside, indoor and food allergies. They print a list of all negative, borderline and positive allergens.

The first thing you should do if you suspect an allergy is to eliminate those things your puppy is allergic to. If that is impossible, then you can treat the allergy itself. Skin allergies are treated with cortisone and topical medications to reduce the itch and inflammation. The cortisone blocks the allergic reaction in the deeper layers of the skin. If the reactions are severe, oral or injected cortisone can be given.

If a food allergy is suspected, a bland hypoallergenic diet of lamb and rice is usually used. Very few dogs are allergic to lamb or rice. Many dogs with food allergies will respond quickly to a hypo allergenic diet.

If your veterinarian thinks your puppy is a candidate, an individualized serum can be made up to all those things the puppy is allergic to. This is the only way to actually desensitize your dog to the things it's allergic to. The idea is that if your vet injects small amounts of the allergens over time (months), your puppy will slowly become desensitized to them. It's the same way allergists treat people who have allergies. This is a commitment in time and money. Allergy shots don't work for months, and they require frequent, regular visits to your vet. Usually the shots start weekly and end monthly. They can continue for years. But for people reluctant to use cortisone and who want a cure instead of just treating the symptoms, this is an option. The prognosis is generally *fair* to *good*, depending on severity.

Cuts and Scrapes

All puppies eventually cut and scrape themselves. If the wound is only superficial, minimal care is needed. Look for the following signs:

- There is only a faint white line on the skin, no gaping wound.
- Instead of bleeding, there is only an ooze of straw-colored fluid (serum).
- There may be hair loss without injury to the skin.
- There is minimal redness and puffiness around the cut. It would be wise to treat superficial cuts and scrapes with basic first aid at home. If you are not sure of the severity of the wound, call your veterinarian and describe the cut. Your vet will want to know:
- How deep is the wound? Can you see the tissues under the skin?
- Is it bleeding, and how hard—just an ooze or dripping?
- Have you attempted any first aid? The procedure we use for treating superficial cuts and scrapes is to wash the area twice daily with hydrogen peroxide and pat dry with a tissue or gauze. Follow with an antibiotic skin ointment. Apply only a thin film, as any excess will prompt the dog to lick it off, which defeats the purpose. If you can cover the wound with a light dressing or bandage, do so.

Warning signs that the wound requires further professional attention are these:

- There is bleeding through the bandage.
- A pus discharge starts a couple of days later, indicating infection.
- There is a foul infectious odor coming from the wound or bandage.
- The wound is in a place that could leave an unwanted scar.

These signs tell you your first aid attempts are inadequate for the wound. A veterinarian may choose oral systemic antibiotics, wound flushing and debridement (removal of dead tissue), or sutures to close a deep laceration. Don't wait too long to seek further help. A superficial infection can develop into a deep one in a matter of a few days. Certain deep infections of flesh are called *gangrene*. Once gangrene sets in, the tissue is usually lost forever, and removal or amputation may be necessary. The prognosis is *very good* for superficial scrapes and cuts as long as they're treated promptly.

Lick Granulomas and Calluses

Both of these afflictions are thickenings of the skin. They have a leathery appearance, are devoid of hair, may be ulcerated and bleed, and are usually round or oblong. That's where the similarity ends. We will discuss each separately, as they have different causes and treatments.

Lick Granuloma

Other names for this are *lick sore* and *acral lick granuloma*. These are self-inflicted sores on the extremities of short-coated dogs. I have seen them on the front legs below the elbow (especially near the wrist joint), and below the knee on the hind legs (especially near the hock joint). What starts these dogs licking at their legs is not totally known. Some speculate that the dogs do it out of boredom. Others say it starts with an itch, like from a bug bite. I feel it is a combination of both. If something itches the dog, and it has the time and opportunity to lick at the spot all day long, a lick sore will develop. The more the dog licks at that spot, the larger and more irritated it gets. So the dog licks even more. It's a vicious cycle.

The size of these lick sores can be from dime- to quarter-sized. They are devoid of hair on the top, raised, thickened, round, often ulcerated in the center and painful to the touch. The skin thickens as a protective response to the constant, irritating licking. In other words, the dog is actually creating this problem due to its instinctive licking mechanism to heal itself. The problem with these cases is that the licking behavior becomes neurotic and/or obsessive. If these dogs simply left their sores alone, they would heal in a matter of a few weeks.

Following is a list of methods I have used to attempt to cure lick sores. They are listed from the easiest to the most complicated. Not all have worked in every case. It may take some trial and error to find the best technique for the individual patient.

- Covering with a bandage to keep the puppy from licking
- Topical anti-inflammatory lotions, which may contain cortisone
- Topical antibiotic ointments
- Systemic antihistamine medications
- Systemic cortisone medications
- Allergy testing and shots
- Elizabethan collar to keep dog from licking
- Muzzling puppy to keep from licking
- Surgical removal of sore

A combination of the preceding techniques may prove most beneficial. Don't hesitate to ask your vet which ones may help your puppy. Some veterinarians are trying to treat this problem with Prozac, the human depression-disorder drug. The prognosis is *good*, as this condition is more annoying than

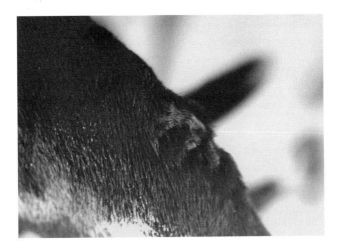

An example of a lick granuloma.

life-threatening. But it is one of the most frustrating conditions to treat, so hang in there!

Callus

Calluses are thickened layers of skin that develop over bony points—typically, the elbow and hock. Calluses are common in large and giant breed dogs over fifty pounds in weight. The constant pressure of the dog lying on these bony joint protuberances causes the skin to become dry, thickened, white, hairless and flaky—protective measures of the body. Calluses are unsightly but of little health consequence. They are identical to the calluses we get on the bottom of our feet. Generally, they require no treatment other than padding the floor where the dog sleeps to relieve the pressure on the callus. Applying a skin moisturizer, like petroleum jelly, can help prevent the callus from cracking. In severe cases, the callus will crack and bleed. Occasionally they become secondarily infected. There can even be water buildup in the callus. This can be painful and may require surgical draining. I do not recommend surgical removal of the callus, as there are many complications, and a new callus usually forms in its place. I have the owner warm-compress the callus, pad the joint, place pads on the floor and give antibiotics to guard against infection. The prognosis is *good*.

Histiocytoma

This is a common skin tumor of young dogs under one year of age. Short-coated dogs are more prone. Histiocytomas are almost always benign (meaning noncancerous). They are the size of a dime or nickel and occur

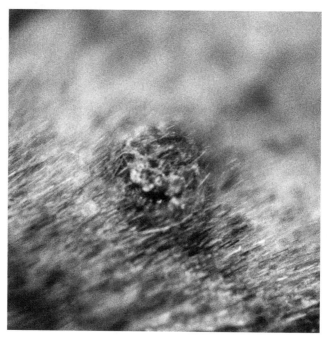

A histiocytoma is a common skin tumor of dogs under one year of age. They occur mainly on the legs and trunk.

mainly on the legs and trunk. They have no hair on them, and are light in color and no deeper than the skin. They can itch, so many puppies lick at them, causing them to bleed and ulcerate.

If left untreated, most will dry up and fall off within several months. Most owners request their removal before that, as these nodules are unsightly. The tumors are easily excised (removed surgically) under a local anesthesic. They are not to be worried about and are more a cosmetic problem than anything else. The prognosis is *good*.

Viral Warts (Papillomatosis)

This infectious disease is caused by the *Papillomavirus* and causes benign wart-like growths on the skin of young puppies. It incubates for thirty days. The warts are grayish in color, and rough and cauliflower-like in appearance. They are found in clusters and can occur in the mouth, ears, eyes, and throat, and on the lips and muzzle. The warts are unsightly and can be dangerous if in the mouth or throat as they can block the throat, making swallowing or breathing difficult. These warts are often self-limiting, which means they may spontaneously resolve on their own within several months. Most owners don't want to wait that long. Treatment is required for warts in the throat.

They are treated with surgical excision, cryosurgery (frozen), electrosurgery (vaporized) or chemicals (burned off). Since these can be more than cosmetic, treatment should be started early. The prognosis is *fair* to *good*.

Autoimmune Skin Disease (Pemphigus)

An autoimmune disease is one in which the body turns against itself for reasons not completely known. Dogs with this ailment mount an immune response against their own skin. This causes inflammation, redness, blistering, bleeding, ulceration and exfoliation of the skin. All this takes time to happen, usually weeks to months. The skin of these dogs literally sloughs off. It is a horrible and, luckily, quite rare disease that can be life-threatening. These dogs look as if they have second- and third-degree burns.

There are several different forms of pemphigus: *pemphigus vegetans*, characterized by tumor wart–like growths along with the skin lesions; *pemphigus vulgaris*, characterized by lesions of the mouth, lips and genitals; and *pemphigus foliaceus*, the most common form, which is characterized by sloughing skin of the face, nose, ears, legs and paws. There are crusting, flaking, ulceration and oozing of the skin, and deep sores. Diagnosis is made via skin biopsy. In fact, biopsy is the only way to confirm this

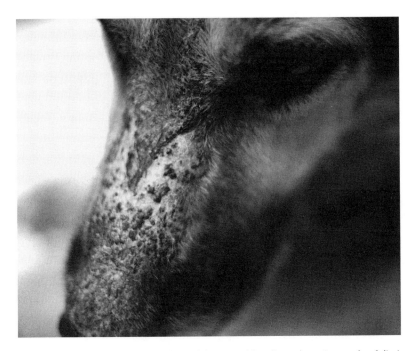

Pemphigus causes inflammation, redness, blistering, bleeding, ulceration and exfoliation of the skin. It is caused by the body turning against itself.

diagnosis. What complicates it is that other skin diseases such as deep pyoderma, burns, other autoimmune diseases, bacterial infections, fungal infections, mange and cancer can look very similar. A biopsy can distinguish among these. Since secondary bacterial infection is common, the biopsy might identify both pemphigus and a secondary bacterial pyoderma.

Pemphigus is not easy to treat. Since the immune system is attacking its own body, the dog has to fight against itself. Immunosuppressive drugs are crucial, the most common being cortisone. Others would include certain chemotherapy drugs. Broad-spectrum antibiotics are often given concurrently. The owner must understand that these drugs aren't curing anything, but merely suppressing the body's ability to attack itself. Because many of these cases can be fatal without these drugs, however, it is a trade-off. The prognosis for most pemphigus cases is *guarded* to *poor*.

Eye, Ear and Throat Diseases

This is a large group of diseases that affect the eyelids, conjunctiva (tissues around the eye), eyeball, ear flap, ear canal, throat and tonsils.

Diseases of the Eyelids and Conjunctiva

Inflammation of the eyelids and conjunctiva can be split into three groups: infectious, immune-mediated and glandular. *Infectious* means that an infectious agent is causing disease to the tissues. *Immune-mediated* means that the dog's body is reacting to something, but not to infectious agents. (The most common immune-mediated inflammation is an allergy.) *Glandular* refers to problems of the hair follicles and oil glands of the eyelids, namely the meibomian and Zeis glands. The three different groups of eyelid disorders are mites (*Demodex* and *Sarcoptes*, full descriptions of which are found in Chapter 3); ringworm fungus (*Microsporum* or *Trichophyton* fungi); and bacterial (*Staphylococcus* is the most common).

Group I: Infectious Agents That Cause Eyelid Disease

This section deals with mites, ringworm fungus and bacteria.

Mites. A full description of mites that infect puppies is found in Chapter 3. The mite that is most often seen around the eyes is demodectic mange.

Ringworm Fungal Infection of the Eyelid. The two fungi that can infect skin are *Microsporum* and *Trichophyton*. They don't just infect the eyelids, but any part of the skin. They are very contagious when

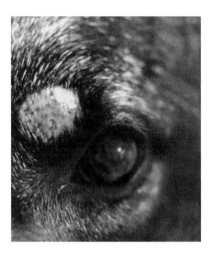

Ringworm is not a worm at all, but a fungal infection that affects the skin, causing redness, itching, hair loss and crusting.

contact with the infected hair occurs. These fungi grow outside during the late fall and into winter. Animals become infected by contacting another animal with the fungus or its contaminated fur. Many wild animals harbor these fungi. Cats are a common source of infection, as many cats become immune to it but carry it on their fur. The fungus causes a localized skin reaction of redness, itching, hair loss and crusting. This often occurs in a circular lesion, hence the name "ringworm." When this occurs on the eyelids, it is usually very noticeable. The fungus creeps to other areas of the head, muzzle and ears.

Diagnosis is made in one of two ways. First, the veterinarian inspects the fur under a black light, which causes the fungus to fluoresce a bright green color. This is not the most accurate means of diagnosing ringworm, as not all species of fungus fluoresce. The second, more accurate means of diagnosing ringworm is a fungal culture. A few hairs from the infected area are plucked and placed on a special media growth plate, which encourages fungal growth. If there is fungus, there will be a significant growth within ten to fourteen days at room temperature. The type of fungus can be identified by the appearance and color of the growth in the eyes of an experienced bacteriologist.

There are several ways of treating fungal infections. One is daily topical application of antifungal creams on the lesions if the lesions are few and localized. The active ingredient in these antifungal creams is miconazole 2 percent, the same ingredient in many over-the-counter athlete's foot treatments (athlete's foot being another fungal infection of people). If the lesions are widespread and severe, oral antifungal medication is used. Your veterinarian may choose a combination of topical as well as oral treatments.

Ringworm fungus is contagious to people, especially children. Washing hands, vacuuming up all dog hair, washing bedding and generally being conscious of hygiene can prevent the spread of fungus. Please consult your doctor if you suspect you've gotten your puppy's ringworm. I've had it three times. The prognosis is generally *fair* to *good*, since most cases of ringworm resolve on their own within a few months.

Bacterial Infections of the Eyelids and Conjunctiva. The bacteria most often cultured from most skin infections is *Staphylococcus*, notorious in skin infections in almost all species of animals. If the infection involves the hair follicles and causes small whiteheads, we call this *folliculitis* or *impetigo*. If the infection involves the tissues around the eye, we call it *conjunctivitis*.

The eyes become swollen and red; pus may exude from open sores; there may be whiteheads; itching may occur; and the conjunctiva may be red and swollen closed. Fortunately, the eyeball itself is usually unharmed. Diagnosis is made by clinical observation of the patient, as well as by taking a bacterial culture of the discharge. Make sure a sensitivity is also done as part of the culture, as *Staphylococcus* bacteria are resistant to many common antibiotics.

Treatment of bacterial eyelid infections and conjunctivitis is accomplished with frequent washings of the eyelid, warm compresses to enhance healing, topical antibiotic ointments to the eyelids (the use of an ophthalmic preparation is advised because most puppies get the ointment in their eyes when rubbing), triple antibiotic ophthalmic ointments in the eye and oral antibiotics. As mentioned previously, make sure the veterinarian chooses one that was proven to be sensitive to the bacteria on the sensitivity report. The prognosis is *good*.

Group 2: Immune Mediated Disorders That Cause Eyelid and Conjunctiva Disease

This group includes allergic reactions (see the section on allergic dermatitis/ atopy for details), autoimmune disease (see the section on pemphigus for details) and hypersensitivity to *Staphylococcus* bacteria (see the section on puppy strangles for details).

Group 3: Problems of the Glands of the Eyelids

Here we look at *chalazion*, an enlargement of the meibomian gland; and the *stye*, an infection of the eyelash hair follicle and its Zeis gland.

> **Chalazion.** This is an enlargement of the *meibomian gland* of the eyelid, an oil gland that secretes a white sebum material that helps lubricate the eye. If the duct become blocked, the gland becomes overfilled and distended. The swelling is observed from the external margin of the eyelid. The swelling should not be painful. Gentle pressure can be applied to encourage drainage. Treatment consists of soaking the lump with warm water and applying an ophthalmic ointment three times daily in hopes of opening the duct. If this procedure fails, the gland can be lanced and the material scooped out or surgically removed from the margin. The prognosis is *good*.

> **Stye.** This is a bacterial infection of the hair follicle of the eyelashes and an oil gland called the *gland of Zeis*. These are red, swollen, painful lumps at the eyelid margin. There can be a pus discharge. The puppy often rubs and paws at the irritation. Treatment consists of soaking the swelling with warm water and applying an ophthalmic ointment three times daily. Oral antibiotics are indicated in severe cases. Gentle pressure can be applied to encourage drainage. The prognosis is *good*.

Diseases of the Eyeball

Horner's Syndrome

This is a neurological disorder that comes from a blunt blow to the eye, trauma to the neck or pressure behind the eye. Another possibility is a mild stroke. Some dogs are prone to blood flow disturbances of their inner and middle ears. This occurs more in geriatric dogs. When certain neural pathways are disrupted, a collection of symptoms occur as described here:

- The eyeball is sunken in its socket.
- The pupil is smaller on the affected side than on the other side.
- The nictitans membrane (the third eyelid) comes up and covers half of the eye.
- Atrophy of the facial muscles occurs on the affected side.

Most of Horner's syndrome in young dogs is brought on by trauma to the eye or that side of the face. Most trauma-induced cases spontaneously resolve on their own as the nerve pathways are re-established. This process can take several weeks. Time is the best remedy for this ailment. Anti-inflammatory drugs such as cortisone can help reduce the swelling of the disrupted nerves, if given systemically. If the condition does not improve with time, your veterinarian will have to check for other causes such as cancer or abscess behind the eye. The prognosis is *fair*.

Corneal Ulcers

The *cornea* is the multilayered transparent covering of the eyeball that we see through. If there is any disruption to the integrity of these layers, an ulcer will develop. Think of a corneal ulcer as an erosion, or pothole, in the cornea. The most common cause is trauma to the eye. A scratch from a cat's claw or low branch can do it. Another common cause is an infection of the eye, also know as conjunctivitis. Certain infections of the tissues that surround the eye can also cause disease of the cornea, with corneal meltdown, leaving a large ulcer.

The symptoms of a corneal ulcer are excess tearing, redness and swelling, squinting and a discoloration of part the cornea.

If the ulceration or extent of the damage is only superficial, healing is usually rapid (with proper treatment). If the ulcer is deeper, involving the deeper layers of the cornea, aggressive therapy may be required. Therefore, it is important to evaluate the depth of the damage. Corneal ulcers are diagnosed by placing an ophthalmic stain in the eye. The vet places a drop of the brilliant green stain in the eye in question, then rinses it out with eyewash. Where the top layers of the cornea are eroded off, the stain will stick. The veterinarian can then visualize where the ulcer is. The ulcer actually fluoresces green. This procedure is called *fluorescent staining*. The vet can also get an idea of how deep the ulcer is.

Treatment depends on how deep the ulcers are. Superficial scratches are treated with a triple ophthalmic antibiotic ointment applied three times daily. Deep ulcers are treated a bit more aggressively, sometimes requiring eyedrops to reduce the pain and associated muscle spasms. The eye may need to be sutured shut so that the conjunctiva, or third eyelid, acts like a natural bandage. Also available are medications that help slow down the melting of the cornea by bacterial enzymes. A combination of all these techniques may be needed. *Never use any medications that contain cortisone in cases of corneal ulcers; they inhibit healing and can make corneal ulcers worse.*

The danger with any corneal ulcers is that the deeper they get, the more chance of them eating through the cornea and rupturing the eyeball. Obviously, at that point there is a real risk of permanent blindness and loss of the eye. All breeds are susceptible to corneal ulcers, but those

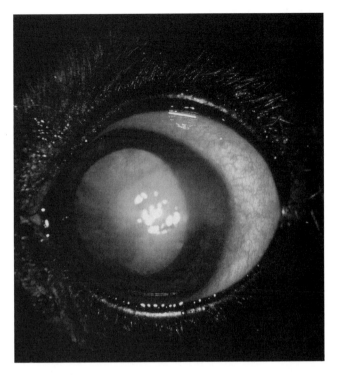

A corneal ulcer, like this one, is a sort of erosion in the cornea caused by trauma or infection. *Dr. M. Neaderland*

breeds with short pushed-in faces with bulging prominent eyes are most prone. With prompt care, superficial ulcers carry a *good* prognosis, while the prognosis for deeper ulcers is only *guarded* to *fair*.

Proptosis

This means displacement of the eyeball out of its socket and happens following trauma to the eye—for example, in a car accident or dog fight. The globe of the eye will actually hang out of its socket. As awful as this looks, the eye may still be saved. In *brachycephalic* breeds (those with short pushed-in faces, like the Pekingese or Shih Tzu), the eyes "pop out" easily and can be just as easily replaced. People should not attempt this themselves; rather, they should seek professional help quickly. On their way to the vet's, they can keep the eye moist with warm water or saline eye wash. An easy way to do this is to place a damp warm washcloth over the dangling eye. Apply gentle even pressure so as to keep the globe from swaying. The veterinarian will have to suture the globe back in the socket by sewing the eye closed. The sutures stay in for several weeks. Depending on the amount of trauma, how long the eye was out of the socket, whether the eye dried out, and whether surrounding tissues were damaged, the eye may not be able to be saved. The prognosis is *guarded* for vision in that eye.

Uveitis

This is defined as an inflammation of the inside structures of the eye, usually involving the iris, inner lining of the eye, and lens attachments. The symptoms are a red, bloodshot eye; pain and pressure within the eye; swollen, red tissues surrounding the eye; a small pupil; cloudy fluid and specks floating in the eye; excess tearing; and blood in the eye.

Causes of uveitis include trauma to the eye, bacterial infections, certain parasites and canine hepatitis. Trauma is the most common cause. A deep corneal ulcer can lead to uveitis, as well as other injuries to the cornea. Other conditions appear similar to uveitis, making the diagnosis tricky.

Treating uveitis is not as complicated as diagnosing it. The main key in treating these cases is to reduce the inflammation inside the eye. Cortisone drugs are best at this. They can be administered in four different ways: as topical ophthalmic drops or ointment; as injections into the conjunctival tissues surrounding the eye; as oral systemic cortisone and/or other anti-inflammatory drugs; or as pain relievers, such as atropine ophthalmic drops, which dilate the pupil.

These cases must be treated aggressively, or the dog runs a distinct risk of the retina detaching, which causes blindness in that eye. Every day the eye has a raging inflammation, the prognosis worsens. Therefore, the prognosis ranges from *guarded* to *poor* for retaining vision.

Retinal Detachment

This is a common sequel to uveitis (described previously) and trauma to the head or eye. Retinal detachment is when the *retina* (the lining of the back of the eyeball that detects the light coming through the lens) separates from the back wall of the eye. A normal retina is essential for normal vision. This is a common ailment of prizefighters who are chronically sustaining head injury from boxing. This condition is easily diagnosed with an eye exam given by a veterinarian. Unfortunately, little treatment is available for this condition, and blindness is inevitable. The prognosis is *poor* for vision in that eye.

Dry Eye (Keratoconjunctivitis Sicca or KCS)

Dry eye is a condition in which the puppy doesn't produce enough tears to keep its eye moist. KCS is the most common eye affliction of dogs. It should be

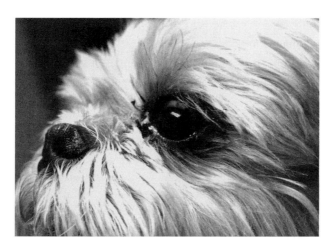

Dry eye, or Keratoconjunctivits Sicca (KCS), is the most common eye affliction of dogs.

suspected anytime there is a chronically red eye with an ocular discharge. A constant flow of tears naturally moistens the cornea with every blink of the eye. If there is a deficiency of tears, the cornea will dry out. The body makes a desperate attempt to moisten the cornea by secreting a thick, yellow pus discharge. This in no way substitutes for tears, but it's the only thing it can do. Other symptoms of KCS include corneal ulceration, a red inflamed eye, squinting, pawing at the eye, a brown film over the cornea, a dull dry cornea and a thick yellow discharge that quickly returns even if you wipe it away often.

Causes of KCS are varied and include breed predilections such as dogs with prominent eyes (Pekingese, Bulldog, Cocker Spaniel), dogs that have had their cherry eye (gland of the third eyelid) surgically removed, eye trauma and generalized dehydration.

Diagnosis is made by measuring the amount of tears the dog produces in a specified time frame. The most popular of these tests is called the *Schirmer Tear Test*. In this test, a strip of paper is placed in the corner of the puppy's eye so that it can absorb the tears. After one minute, the wet part of the strip is measured. Normal dogs will have at least seven millimeters of wet strip. Less than that indicates low tear production.

Treatment is easy with artificial tear medications available over the counter in ophthalmic drops or ointment. They are to be applied in the eye several times daily. *Without the tear replacements, the eye will dry out and go blind.* Recently a drug has been approved for use in dogs which stimulates natural tear production. This drug is called Cyclosporine and is available for veterinary use as an ointment that is applied twice daily. It has shown promising results. There are surgical procedures that can be done which transplant a salivary duct to the eye so that the dog literally drools into its eye. I personally don't do this procedure. I've seen at least as many failures as successes. Considering the new medications and lubricants available, I see little need for this questionable surgery. The prognosis is *guarded* to *fair* for normal vision.

Diseases of the Ears

Ear Mites

A full description of these little mites that live in the ear canals of dogs is found in Chapter 3.

Yeast Otitis Externa

Yeast is the budding form of fungus. A certain amount of yeast normally lives in the ears of dogs; if water gets trapped in the outer ear canal, the yeast will start to flourish. This happens during swimming and bathing. The yeasts that thrive in a dog's ear canal are *Candida albicans* and *Malassezia*.

The symptoms of yeast otitis externa are: head shaking; scratching at the ears; a very sour, curdled odor from the ears; red, inflamed, and intensely itchy ears; a brown, crusty accumulation in the ear canal; self-induced abrasions from the dog scratching its ear; and a dark brown, waxy discharge from the ears.

The diagnosis is easily made during a physical exam by your veterinarian. The characteristic sour smell; copious brown, waxy discharge; and intense itching clinch the diagnosis. If there is still a question, a culture can be performed. *Be aware that a bacterial culture will not grow yeast. Therefore, if yeast is suspected, a fungal culture should be done instead.*

Treatment is usually threefold. First, a thorough cleaning of the ears must be done to remove all debris and infectious material from the ear canal. This should be done by a veterinarian. A cleaner specifically designed for dog ears should be used. Most have a ceruminolytic agent (which breaks up wax), and some contain an antiseptic to kill yeast. Next, topical anti-yeast ointments are squirted into the ear canal once or twice daily for seven to ten days. Then, if the infection is severe, the vet may prescribe oral anti-yeast drugs as well.

The breeds most prone to yeast ear infections are those with long, floppy ear flaps that hang down and cover the opening to the ear canal. If you have a puppy that is developing a chronic ear problem, you may want to follow some of the preventive measures described in the section about bacterial otitis externa. The prognosis is usually *fair* to *good* with prompt treatment.

Any dog that swims regularly or is bathed frequently runs a high risk of getting water down the ear canal, which predisposes the dog to yeast otitis externa.

Bacterial Otitis Externa

Bacterial ear canal infections come in two varieties: pus-producing and non–pus-producing. Even the novice owner can identify these infections. In the *pus-producing* kind, there is a yellowish-green discharge from the ear canal and usually a foul odor. The *non–pus-producing* infections are harder to spot at first. There is no discharge, but there is an odor, and the ear is every bit as red and inflamed as in the other form. Whether an infection is pus-producing or not depends on the bacteria growing, as some stimulate pus and others don't. Certain bacteria commonly reside in the ear canal. If the conditions are right for the bacteria to multiply (dark, damp and warm, with reduced air flow), there will be a flourish of bacterial growth, resulting in enough to cause disease. We call this an overgrowth of bacteria. The bacteria that commonly reside in and can potentially infect ears are *Staphylococcus*, *Pseudomonas*, *Proteus* and *Streptococcus*. A veterinarian usually needs to culture the ear canal to get an identification. Also, a sensitivity report should be done. This is part of the culture report, and it lists the appropriate antibiotics that will kill the specific bacteria grown in the culture. The symptoms of otitis externa are: head shaking; scratching at the ears; an infectious odor from the ears; a pus discharge if the infection is suppurative; red, inflamed, painful ears; a crusty accumulation in the ear canal; and self-induced abrasions from the dog scratching its ear.

Diagnosis of otitis externa is made by a veterinarian. A physical exam will reveal the changes seen in the ear canal, and the culture will identify the bacterial agent. Treatment is similar to that for a yeast condition, except the drugs attack bacteria.

Some cases of otitis externa become chronic or prolonged. If you have a puppy that is developing a chronic ear problem, you may want to follow some of these preventive measures:

- Keep the hairs short around the ears. This allows the air to get into the external ear canal. Circulating air prohibits bacterial and yeast growth.
- Clean out the external ear canals as often as necessary to keep them clean. This may mean once a month or twice a week, depending on the breed of puppy. The ear canal should be pink and clean. A dark

brown, waxy discharge could indicate an ear problem. See Chapter 4 for preventive health care of the ears and proper cleaning techniques.

- If your puppy is a breed that has a lot of hair in its ear canals, have the hair plucked regularly to help in the general hygiene of the puppy's ears.
- Try to limit the amount of swimming your puppy does. When it swims, water often gets in its ears, which leads to yeast and bacterial ear infections. If you cannot restrict the swimming, then rinse out your dog's ears with an antiseptic ear cleaner after each swim; this will reduce chances of infection.
- Place cotton in the ears of your puppy before giving it a bath. This keeps the water out.
- If your puppy has been diagnosed with an ear infection, whether it be ear mites, bacteria or yeast, make sure you finish giving the appropriate ear medication. If you stop too soon, a relapse could occur.

Ear Flap Trauma and Hematoma

Breeds with long, drooping ear flaps are most susceptible to trauma. Ear-flap trauma could result from a dog getting into dog fights, being hit by a car, having the ear caught in a door or stepped on, being bitten by flies, snagging on wire fences or getting a bad cropping job.

The trauma can range from a superficial scrape or wound to a full-thickness laceration or puncture. Clearly, the superficial scrapes are not serious. The deeper, full-thickness cuts and punctures require veterinary care. They bleed an awful lot and usually require stitches. Here are a few things to keep in mind if an ear flap trauma happens to your puppy: 1) ear flap wounds bleed a lot, so follow first aid tips in Chapter 5 to control the bleeding and learn how to stop it; 2) if the puncture is full thickness through the ear flap, it will require suturing. Many ear wounds leave permanent ear notches and disfigurement.

Aural Hematoma

In this condition, a blood vessel in the ear flap between the skin and the inner ear cartilage bleeds, leading to a large blood clot (*hematoma*) in the ear flap. This egg-sized swelling is very noticeable to the owner and painful to the puppy. The diagnosis is very easy to make. If your puppy has a sudden large swelling of the ear flap that is sensitive to the touch, it's most likely an aural hematoma. The afflicted ear hangs lower than the other, normal side; and the puppy, because of the discomfort, shakes its head a lot. These ears must be treated; otherwise there will be permanent disfiguring of the ear flap. After a few months, the blood clot starts to organize and harden. This causes the ear flap to crinkle and become cauliflower-like.

Treatment of aural hematomas is surgery. At the very least, the blood clot should be drained. This can be done by a veterinarian with an aspirate needle. If the veterinarian aspirates only the hematoma and does not remove the solidified blood clot, the ear flap often fills up again. For those reasons, the more effective treatment is for the veterinarian to lance open the hematoma; remove the solids; and then suture the ear skin to the cartilage, leaving a small drainage hole or port open. This keeps the ear flap flat, and the opening prevents it from filling up again while it heals. The sutures stay in place for several weeks. The hole in the center heals on its own by the time the sutures come out. These cases should be placed on antibiotics for the duration of the healing. The prognosis is generally *good*.

Diseases of the Throat

Tonsillitis

This is the most common ailment of the throat of young dogs. Young puppies are always putting things in their mouths that they shouldn't, from stuff in the cat's litterbox to their own stools. They pull things out of the garbage and lick things off the floor. Many of these items introduce bacteria into the throats of puppies who haven't yet developed a resistance to them. The bacteria inhabit the back of the throat where the tonsillar lymph nodes are. Once these become infected, the puppy suffers a sore throat. The tonsils become swollen, red and painful. At this point, the owners usually notice that the puppy won't eat, or tries to and can't swallow. It may make gagging noises and seem lethargic. There may be a foul odor from the mouth and a concurrent fever.

The diagnosis is made by palpating the large, egg-sized glands in the neck just behind the angle of the jaw. Inspection of the tonsils reveals the source of the infection. Your veterinarian will probably opt for a throat culture to identify the bacteria. The bacterium to be most worried about is *Streptococcus*. Certain strains of this bacterium have been known to be contagious to people, and vice versa. In fact, I have gotten calls from pediatricians requesting me to culture a new puppy for *Streptococcus* because the children in the house are infected. The pediatricians were trying to identify the source. I recommend that if your children are suffering from chronic "strep" throat infections, have a throat culture done on your puppy.

Treatment is to start antibiotics. If a sensitivity report was done with the culture, it will tell the vet which antibiotics are appropriate for that specific bacterium. A minimum of a seven- to ten-day course is needed to reduce the chances of a relapse. It is very rare that the tonsils need to be surgically removed. This practice is no longer in fashion.

Respiratory Diseases

The respiratory tract is that part of the body that allows breathing. It starts at the nose and includes the sinuses, larynx, trachea (windpipe), bronchi, lungs, diaphragm and rib cage. Each breath is a complex series of muscle contractions that leads to air being drawn into the body. Once the air enters the nasal passages, it is filtered, warmed and humidified by the nasal passages and the sinuses before it enters the lungs. Fine dirt particles are also filtered out before the air passes into the lungs. Once in the lungs, the air undergoes two transfers: 1) Oxygen from the air is absorbed into the blood flowing through the lung capillaries, and 2) carbon dioxide in the blood flowing through the lungs is transferred into the expired air that is expelled when exhaled.

If any one of these processes doesn't happen right on cue, breathing difficulties will result. This section starts with the nose and sinuses, and follows along down the tract to end with diseases of the lungs.

Rhinitis and Upper Respiratory Infection (URI)

Rhinitis means inflammation of the nasal passages. A nose can become swollen and stuffy because of viral rhinitis, bacterial rhinitis or allergic rhinitis.

> **Viral Rhinitis.** Literally dozens of rhinitis viruses can infect puppies. They all are contagious via droplets that spew out of a sneezing dog's nose. The incubation period of most of these viruses is from three days to a week. Sneezing, a clear watery nasal discharge, runny eyes, low-grade fever and sensitivity to light are the most common symptoms. *In viral rhinitis, there is always a watery nasal discharge.*
>
> The most common viruses that infect a dog's upper respiratory tract are the canine distemper virus, canine adenovirus type-2 virus and canine parainfluenza virus. All are discussed thoroughly in Chapter 2, "All About Vaccines."
>
> Treatment of viral rhinitis is directed toward drying up the nasal passages. Decongestants help reduce the runny nose, and antibiotics are also given if secondary bacterial infection is a consideration. The important thing is to realize that these dogs are contagious to other dogs for at least a week. Most puppies do fine, and it's just a matter of time before they're recovered. The prognosis of most viral rhinitis (except for canine distemper) is *good.*

Bacterial Rhinitis. Bacterial rhinitis is very similar to viral rhinitis except that it's accompanied by a fever and a thick yellow nasal discharge. The bacteria that inhabit the canine nasal passages are usually either *Staphylococcus* or *Streptococcus* species. Your veterinarian will probably want to culture the pus discharge in an attempt to identify the bacteria. If a sensitivity report is run with the culture, the appropriate antibiotics will be listed. Amoxicillin is a favorite amongst many vets. If there is much congestion of the nose, room humidifiers and decongestants may help. The danger of bacterial rhinitis is the possibility of it spreading into the sinuses, causing a sinusitis, or down into the bronchi, causing a bronchitis. Therefore, the prognosis of an uncomplicated bacterial rhinitis is *fair* to *good*. The prognosis worsens as the infection spreads.

Allergic Rhinitis and Airborne Irritants. Allergies are the number-one cause of a watery, itchy nose in dogs. Those that affect the nose are virtually the same as those that affect the eyes. The nose becomes runny and red. There may be sneezing or itching in the nose, so the puppy rubs its nose along the floor or with his paws. In severe cases, there can be nosebleeds. *As in the case of viral rhinitis, the nasal discharge will be clear and watery, making it difficult to differentiate between the two.*

Diagnosis is made by observing the symptoms in different situations. For example, maybe your puppy has a sneezing spell every time it goes in the basement where it's dusty and there's mold growing on the walls. Mold and dust are two common allergies of dogs. Perhaps your puppy only has a runny nose and itchy eyes from late August to October, the ragweed season. Many allergies are seasonal. In fact, the seasonal symptoms help identify the allergy. The complete diagnosis and treatment of allergies is given in Chapter 4: "Care of the Eyelids, Conjunctiva and Eyeball." The only difference is that decongestants can be used for a runny nose.

Sinusitis

Sinusitis is defined as the inflammation of the lining (mucosa) of the sinus cavities. Think of sinusitis as a progression and continuation of rhinitis. We all have sinuses. Dogs have bigger sinuses proportionally than people do. Sinuses are open cavities in the skull where the air breathed in or out must pass. In the sinuses, the air is warmed or cooled, and humidified. Fine dirt particles are filtered out before the air passes into the lungs. The sinuses are lined by a moist lining of tissue called a *mucosa*. It stays wet and glistening. If this lining becomes irritated, inflamed or swollen, sinusitis occurs.

The symptoms of sinusitis are a congested sound when the dog breathes in or out; sneezing; a low-grade fever; a thick, yellow nasal discharge, or post-nasal drip into the back of the throat; gagging, choking or coughing; and squinting of the eyes.

The same causes of rhinitis can cause a sinusitis: viral, bacterial or allergic. The diagnosis and treatment are the same as well. Please refer to the section called "Rhinitis and Upper Respiratory Infection (URI)" for details. In severe cases, an X ray of the sinuses will show an eroded sinus lining, implying chronic inflammation. Another difference between sinusitis and rhinitis is in the duration of treatment. Cases of sinusitis can take weeks of treatment before alleviation of symptoms. The prognosis also slips a notch in cases of sinusitis, being from *fair* to *guarded*, due to its chronic nature.

Laryngitis

The congenital disorder of laryngeal paralysis was described in Chapter 1. The infectious type of laryngitis is much more common. The causes of infectious laryngitis are the same as those of infectious rhinitis: viral, bacterial and allergic. The respective causes are the same as for rhinitis. The symptoms are slightly different, however, and include gagging and coughing; a change in the tone or an absence of the bark; and stridor, or inspiratory breathing difficulty. Think of laryngitis as a continuation and progression of sinusitis.

Diagnosis is made by a veterinarian listening to the squeaky sounds produced when the puppy tries to bark, and by visualizing the opening to the larynx, called the *epiglottis*. It will appear red and swollen. The treatment and prognosis for infectious laryngitis are the same as for infectious rhinitis.

Bronchitis/Pneumonia

Bronchitis is defined as inflammation of the bronchi, or air passages, of the lungs. The *bronchi* are the tubes that carry the air in and out of the lungs. If their mucosal lining is swollen, inflamed or wet, the efficiency with which they can transport air is compromised, and breathing will suffer. Since the bronchi become narrow and constricted as they branch into the lungs, it doesn't take much congestion to plug them up. *Pneumonia* is the inflammation of the actual lung tissues involved in gaseous transport (oxygen and carbon dioxide). If both bronchitis and pneumonia are present, the condition is called *bronchopneumonia*. This combination of the two is very common.

The causes of bronchopneumonia in the dog are also viral, bacterial and allergic. The most common viruses that cause bronchopneumonia are the Tracheobronchitis virus (kennel cough), described in Chapter 2; the parainfluenza virus; and the adenovirus type-2 virus. These viruses are spread by the coughing of an infected dog. The incubation period is usually several days. The dogs in the immediate area are susceptible (if not vaccinated) and will most likely come down with the disease if there was sufficient exposure.

The common bacterial causative agents are the *Streptococcus, Bordetella bronchiseptica* and *Pasturella* species. They are also spread through the coughing of an infected dog. The incubation period of the bacteria is shorter than for the viruses: about two to five days. Allergic bronchopneumonia is relatively rare in dogs and therefore will not be discussed. Regardless of the cause, the symptoms are virtually the same: coughing, fever, loss of bark, breathing difficulties and wheezing, and noisy lung sounds when breathing.

Diagnosis is made by a veterinarian observing these symptoms and listening to the chest of the dog with a stethoscope. There is also a characteristic breathing pattern that can be visualized during breathing. An X ray of the chest will reveal a typical bronchitis pattern, with thickened bronchial walls and fluid accumulation within or around the bronchi, as well as areas of fluid accumulation within the lung tissues characteristic of pneumonia. A complete blood count will have an elevated white blood cell count, reflecting the infectious nature of the disease.

Treatment includes long-term antibiotics and expectorants, which help bring up the lung congestion. Bronchodilator drugs can be used to help open the congested bronchi. A bacterial culture of the sputum (the stuff that is coughed up) will help identify the appropriate antibiotic for that particular bacteria. Vaporizers used in the room the dog sleeps in can also help loosen the congestion in the chest. Bronchopneumonia can be very serious, even life-threatening in a young puppy. Therefore, it carries a *guarded* prognosis.

Gastrointestinal Diseases

This section is one of the most important for any new puppy owner. All puppies have digestive upsets now and then; in fact, occasional vomiting or diarrhea are normal. This stems from the fact that most puppies eat things they shouldn't, which leads to excess gas, vomiting or diarrhea. The upset should pass as quickly as it comes on. These episodes are of little concern as long as they are infrequent.

The parasitic causes of gastrointestinal disorders were described in Chapter 3. Considering that up to 80 percent of all puppies are born with intestinal parasites (worms), this can account for a high percentage of puppy illness. One of the first things a veterinarian should do for your puppy is to check for worms. Please refer to Chapter 3 if you suspect any parasitic problem in your puppy.

Congenital defects of the intestinal tract were covered in Chapter 1. These include imperforate anus, dysphagia, megaesophagus and persistent right aortic arch.

All of these are defects of the gastrointestinal tract noticed by six months of age. Please refer to that chapter for complete details of these problems.

Common viral gastroenteritis was discussed in Chapter 2. The two viruses detailed are canine parvovirus and canine coronavirus. Both can be very serious. The remaining common gastrointestinal conditions are outlined in the rest of this section. The gastrointestinal tract starts with the mouth and ends with the anus. This section deals mostly with the stomach, intestines, colon and rectum.

Motion Sickness

All of us have taken our puppies and dogs for car rides from time to time. If for no other reason than to go to the vet! What many new puppy owners find is that about ten to fifteen minutes into the ride their puppy starts to salivate, drool, and may dry heave or vomit. The puppy is suffering from motion sickness. The motion of the car is causing the nausea center of the brain to send signals to the stomach to purge itself. Stopping the car will alleviate the symptoms within minutes. If you are planning a trip with your puppy, follow these guidelines:

Motion Sickness Guidelines

1. Don't feed your puppy the morning of the trip.

2. Only give small amounts of water over several hours during the trip so he doesn't drink too much at one time.

3. Use the over-the-counter antimotion sickness drugs available at pharmacies starting one hour before the trip. Ask your veterinarian what dose is appropriate for your puppy.

Vomiting and Inappetence (Gastritis)

Gastritis is defined as an inflammation of the lining of the stomach. Gastritis leads to inappetence and vomiting. *Vomiting* is defined as the forceful expelling of stomach contents through stomach, abdominal muscle and intestinal contractions. Vomiting is very different from *regurgitation*, which is a passive reflux of food out of the esophagus that never made it into the stomach.

Inappetence simply means loss of appetite. Inappetence and vomiting go hand-in-hand. The first thing people notice is that their puppy is quiet and sluggish. This progresses to excess drooling and salivation. Ultimately, the heaving starts. The contractions can seem quite violent at times.

When you first notice the stomach upset, call your veterinarian. He or she will try to determine how serious it is. Obviously, the more frequently and longer it occurs, the worse it is. The duration and severity of the inappetence and vomiting are crucial to determining the cause. Your vet will ask you the following questions:

- When did it start?
- How many times did the puppy vomit today?
- What came up: food, bile, foam, blood?
- What color was the vomit?
- Is the puppy eating or drinking? Is it keeping it down?
- Does the puppy seem sick otherwise? Is it playful or lethargic?
- Can you take its temperature?
- Is there diarrhea also?
- Did your puppy eat anything strange today?
- Is your puppy on any medications?
- Does your puppy eat any household or yard plants?
- Are any of your child's toys missing?
- Has your puppy been checked for internal parasites recently?
- Does your puppy tend to eat objects off the floor?
- Is your puppy out in the sun all day?
- Is your puppy under any unusual stress lately?

Vomiting and gastritis can be from many different causes. Listed here are causes of gastritis followed by a **V**, meaning it causes primarily vomiting; an **I**, meaning inappetence; or both letters.

Causes of Gastritis

- A stuffy nose (dogs like to smell before eating): I
- Any debilitating internal disease: I,V
- Infectious bacterial or viral diseases: I,V
- Infectious gastroenteritis (usually viral): V

continues

Causes of Gastritis *(continued)*

- Certain medications (antibiotics, anti-inflammatory drugs, wormers): I,V

- Constipation (severe): I,V

- Dietary indiscretion (eating something they shouldn't have): V

- Fever: I

- Food poisoning: V

- Gastric ulcers: I,V

- Heat stroke: V

- Ingesting a foreign body: I,V

- Ingesting poisons or poisonous plants: V

- Internal metabolic disorders: I,V

- Internal parasites: I,V
- Overeating: V

- Poor quality food: I,V

- Stress: I

It is very important to get a firm diagnosis in cases of prolonged vomiting or inappetence. Often, this means having diagnostic tests performed to determine the cause. In the event your veterinarian has determined that the gastritis is serious enough to warrant diagnostic measures, you will be asked to bring your puppy into the office for testing. Testing includes barium swallow X rays to identify esophageal problems; blood work-up, including a CBC, chemistry profile, Lyme titer and heartworm test; exploratory surgery to see inside the stomach; a fecal bacterial culture for food poisoning; a fecal digestive analysis to evaluate pancreatic digestive function; a fecal examination for internal parasites; radiographs of the abdomen for foreign bodies; rectal or fecal direct smears for giardiasis; a stomach biopsy to rule out stomach cancer; and a stomach endoscopy to visualize the gastric lining.

Many mild, brief cases of vomiting or loss of appetite are treated with symptomatic therapy. *Symptomatic therapy* is when the doctor treats the symptoms without sometimes knowing what's causing them. This is rarely as effective as treating the cause of the problem, but often it suffices, and the animal recovers. Because it can be so hard to find the cause of vomiting and inappetence, many veterinarians start with symptomatic treatments. These include restricting food and water for eight to twelve hours following a vomiting episode, followed by small amounts of water or a bowl of ice cubes; giving oral antacids or stomach-coating bismuth liquids; replacing drinking water with electrolyte-replacement solutions available at your pharmacy; administering anti-nausea drugs available from your vet; and administering stomach acid inhibitors to reduce nausea. If the symptomatic approach doesn't work, then it's time to go back to basics and get a diagnosis. Severe cases of gastritis require aggressive treatment and sometimes hospitalization.

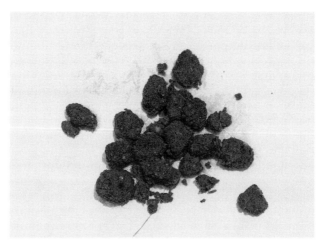

Regurgitated food, which differs from vomit in that it never made it as far as the stomach.

Don't confuse a symptom with a diagnosis. For example, if your puppy is vomiting and you take it to the vet, who says, "Your puppy has gastroenteritis," then you should ask, "From what?" Gastroenteritis is as much a symptom as a diagnosis. It doesn't tell you what is causing the intestinal upset. If your vet is used to managing these cases with symptomatic therapy, you may get the response, "It doesn't really matter what the cause is; we'll treat the puppy for the vomiting anyway." This is all right, as long as both of you realize that the treatment is palliative.

Bloat and Stomach Dilatation-Volvulus

Bloat is a condition in which the stomach becomes overinflated with gas. The abdomen inflates and distends like a balloon within an hour or two. Besides being extremely uncomfortable, this condition can be fatal. It all depends on how distended the stomach becomes. The second part of this disease is the *dilatation-volvulus*, which occurs when, as the stomach distends with gas, it actually twists on itself, shutting off the inflow and outflow pipes. This makes matters critical. All of a sudden, there is no way for the gas to escape. The stomach just keeps filling. This quickly results in cardiac shock and death. In these cases, death can occur quickly in a few hours.

The breeds most predisposed to bloating and dilatation-volvulus are the large and giant dogs with deep chests. The most frequently diagnosed breed is the Great Dane. I have seen it in other large breeds, such as the German Shepherd Dog, Doberman Pinscher, Akita, Mastiff and Irish Wolfhound, to

Differentiation Between Simple Stomach Bloating and Dilatation-Volvulus		
Observation/Test Result	Simple Bloating	Dilatation-Volvulus
Slightly uncomfortable abdomen	Yes	No
Very painful abdomen, hunched over	No	Yes
Excess salivation, drooling, nausea	Yes	Yes
Pale or white mucous membranes	No	Yes
Vomiting with something coming up	Yes	No
Dry heaving with nothing coming up	No	Yes
Evidence of shock	No	Yes
Rapid heart rate and irregular beats	No	Yes
Distended abdomen	Yes	Yes
Rapid breathing	Yes	Yes
Shallow breathing	No	Yes
Thin weak pulses	No	Yes
Concurrent diarrhea	Yes	Yes
Can pass a stomach tube into the stomach	Yes	No
A normal, but distended stomach x ray	Yes	No
X rays show: gas distention, stomach outflow pylorus on top instead of bottom, and a	No	Yes

name a few. Males and females are equally affected. The good news is that although puppies under six months often have bloating, they rarely twist their stomachs and have the dilatation-volvulus component. The causes of bloating and dilatation-volvulus are breed predilection, which means some breeds bloat despite your efforts to prevent it; overeating at one time; drinking a large quantity of water after eating; heavy exercise within an hour after eating; and feeding a poor-quality kibble that expands when wet inside the stomach. The first signs of bloat and or dilatation-volvulus are lethargy and weakness; pale mucous membranes; excessive drooling and salivation; vomiting or dry heaving; a distended, painful abdomen; and hunching over when the puppy stands.

If you notice any of these signs, get to your veterinarian quickly. He or she can identify whether the problem is simply a bloated stomach or the much more serious twisted stomach. This is done by a thorough physical exam and X rays.

Once the diagnosis of either simple bloat or dilatation-volvulus is made, treatment can be started. The two conditions are treated very differently. Only a veterinarian can accurately differentiate between the two.

Treatment of Simple Bloat

Since this condition is not life-threatening, it is not an emergency. Most veterinarians treat these cases and then observe for any signs of progressing to a dilatation-volvulus. The common treatment protocol for a simple bloat may include passing a stomach tube to "pump" and empty the stomach of food, water or gas (decompression); giving antacids orally or through a stomach tube; giving anti-gas liquids orally or through a stomach tube, to break up gas bubbles; and restricting all food and water for twelve hours. The prognosis of uncomplicated bloat is *good*, but your puppy will have a terrible stomachache.

Treatment of Dilatation-Volvulus

The treatment of complicated bloat with dilatation-volvulus is much trickier than that of simple bloat. The timing of emergency care is critical. If the twisted stomach isn't untwisted within a couple of hours, the dog will most likely die. Following are the steps for treating these cases.

Emergency Procedure for Dilatation-Volvulus

1. Immediate intravenous fluid administration with anti-shock cortisone medications.

2. Decompression of the stomach (letting out the gas) to relieve the pressure, which is a strain on the heart. Since the stomach is twisted on itself, the esophagus is twisted shut. This prevents the passage of a stomach tube. The gas is released by a large bore needle placed into the abdomen and through the stomach wall. Once the pressure is relieved, a stomach tube is placed to empty the stomach completely. This greatly helps the survival rate in these cases.

3. Once the pressure is released, abdominal surgery is performed to correct the displaced stomach. The veterinary surgeon needs to untwist the stomach and tack it down so that it can't twist again.

4. The heart must be constantly monitored, as these dogs often have fatal heart arrhythmia during the manipulation of the stomach. Medications are available that can help guard against that.

Even with all this immediate care and surgery, the survival rate is still only about 50 percent. There is a recovery period of weeks, and many postoperative complications arise. The prognosis is *guarded* to *poor*.

Diarrhea and Colitis

Diarrhea is defined as a loose stool; *colitis* is severe diarrhea with straining and, often, bloody stools. When stool material passes too quickly through the colon, there isn't a chance for the water to get absorbed from it. This leads to diarrhea and watery, loose stools. Or, if a dog is on a high-fiber diet, the non-digestible fiber holds water, keeping it from being absorbed and accomplishing the same thing. There are many different types and causes of diarrhea. The most common cause is "dietary indiscretion"—when your dog eats something it shouldn't. Examples of dietary indiscretion are dead animals, other animals' feces, garbage, bars of soap, paper or spoiled food. The following chart lists other causes of diarrhea.

We will describe each group separately to show the differences. Not all diarrhea is the same! Each causative agent produces a slightly different kind of diarrhea.

> **Viral Diarrhea.** The most common viral intestinal infections (which we call enteritis) are canine parvovirus and coronavirus, which were described in detail in Chapter 2. To recap, these are highly contagious viral diseases of dogs that cause a severe inflammation of the intestines, leading to profuse watery and bloody diarrhea. These are always accompanied by fever and, often, vomiting. These puppies quickly dehydrate without supportive care. There is a high mortality rate in young puppies under five months of age.
>
> **Bacterial Diarrhea.** Bacterial infections of the intestines (enteritis) are common in puppies that eat things they shouldn't. Many people classify these as food poisonings. Salmonella is the most common. It is found in bad food, raw chicken and animal feces (especially barnyard animals). These infections may also be accompanied by vomiting,

fever, severe abdominal pains and dark and bloody stools. Antibiotics and supportive care are crucial for treating these patients. These infections are not as contagious as viral enteritis. Since people can become infected with salmonella, great care should be taken not to contaminate human food sources.

Protozoal Diarrhea. The two most common protozoal diarrheas are Giardiasis and Coccidiosis. (Both diseases are fully described in Chapter 3.) These small organisms populate the small and large intestines, causing inflammation and mucus secretion. The puppies generally have soft, mucusy or bloody stools for weeks or months. Giardiasis is common where there are natural water sources where the dog drinks, getting exposure to the protozoa in the water. Wild animal and water bird droppings also contain the infective stage of the protozoa. Many dogs eat bird and wild animal droppings and infect themselves. Coccidiosis is common in breeding kennels where many dogs are housed together. Coccidia is transmitted by infective feces. Treatment for protozoal diseases consists of anti-protozoal drugs. Prevention involves avoiding exposure to outside water sources or wild animal droppings, and good hygiene in a breeding kennel situation.

Parasitic Diarrhea. Internal parasites are perhaps the most common cause of diarrhea in puppies. Studies have shown that up to 80 percent of all puppies born have internal parasites, also called worms. There are several different worms, and each is very different. Complete descriptions are in Chapter 3. Most worms cause a loose, dark, very smelly diarrhea, which can progress to a bloody one. Many other symptoms clue a veterinarian into the diagnosis of internal parasites. Worming medications are available for each type of worm. Therefore, it's important that an accurate diagnosis and identification of the parasite be made.

Autoimmune Diarrhea. Autoimmune and allergic diseases can cause severe diarrhea in dogs. The two disorders most often diagnosed are food allergies and lymphocytic-plasmacytic enteritis. Food allergies occur when a dog eats a food substance to which it's allergic. Lymphocytic-plasmacytic enteritis is a condition in which there is inflammation of the intestinal lining where digestion is impaired. Both of these disorders cause decreased digestion; greasy, light-colored diarrhea; weight loss; and excess flatulence. There is evidence to suggest that some lymphocytic-plasmacytic enteritis of the intestines is caused by food allergies, so there can be some overlap of the two diseases.

The breeds most affected are the German Shepherd Dog and Basenji. Affected puppies are noticeably thin by the age of four to five months. Even though they eat very well, they cannot put on weight. They have greasy, soft, yellow stools. When tested, most of these dogs have food allergies to common components in commercial dog food, whether it be corn, soybean meal or some other food group. Some of these dogs also have a concurrent pancreatic enzyme deficiency requiring enzyme supplementation (see Chapter 1 for details).

The diagnosis is confirmed with an intestinal lining biopsy. Treatment of these cases includes removing the food substance from the dog's diet, supplemental pancreatic enzymes, and cortisone drugs to reduce the inflammation of the intestinal lining, as well as frequent small feedings of a bland diet. An excellent diet for allergic dogs is a lamb-and-rice-formulated food. Very few dogs are allergic to either lamb or rice. Prognosis is generally *fair* to *good*, but these dogs never reach their ideal weight.

Dietary Indiscretion. This means that a puppy eats things it shouldn't. Dogs like grass, plants, paper, soil, upholstery, carpet, floor mats, stool from other animals or themselves, and children's toys. All these things can cause severe diarrhea as they pass through the intestines and lower bowel. If this is the cause, the diarrhea will be brief. As soon as the offending material passes, the diarrhea will resolve on its own. The owner often reports the material coming out of the rectum or seen in the feces. Very little treatment is needed as long as the material passes.

Making a diagnosis for diarrhea is sometimes a complicated task. Tests are usually performed to help rule out certain causes. If the diarrhea only happened once or twice, most veterinarians won't go through the trouble of performing diagnostic tests. In chronic cases of diarrhea, it is imperative to get a firm diagnosis. The chart on page 227 matches causes with the appropriate test.

Regardless of the specific cause of diarrhea, there are some universal treatments that help slow down the passage of stool through the intestines and colon. If your puppy has been diagnosed with one of the specific types of diarrhea described in the chart, follow your veterinarian's treatment suggestions. Occasional diarrhea can be treated by:

- Feeding small meals of a bland diet (chicken and rice, or boiled chopped meat and rice) *three to four times daily*

Common Causes and Types of Diarrhea		
	Causative Agents	**Consistency of Diarrhea**
Viral	Canine Coronavirus	watery and bloody stools
	Canine Parvovirus	watery and bloody stools
	Canine Distemper Virus	watery and bloody stool
Bacterial	Salmonellosis	bloody and dark stools
	Campylobacter	bloody and dark stools
	Shigellosis	bloody and dark stools
Protozoal	Giardiasis	mucous coating on loose stools
	Coccidiosis	mucous coating and bloody stools
Parasitic	Roundworms	loose and foul smelling stools
	Hookworms	loose and foul smelling stools
	Whipworms	watery and bloody stools
Immune-Mediated	Tapeworms	slightly soft stools, rectal itching
	Lymphocytic-Plasmacytic	loose, greasy, yellow stools Enteritis
	Food Allergy Enteritis	loose, greasy, yellow stools

- Giving other bland foods such as cottage cheese, bread, plain yogurt, potato or noodles
- Using anti-diarrhea medications, such as Loperamide, and soothing/coating bismuth liquids
- Giving oral fluids and electrolyte replacement solutions to compensate for water and salt loss
- Using intestinal antibiotics in an attempt to promote digestive bacterial growth and inhibit the "bad" bacteria
- Using *Acidophilus* bacteria (found in active culture yogurt) to aid in digestion

Bloody Diarrhea and Colitis

There are many causes of bloody diarrhea. They are most often infectious, as in viral, bacterial or parasitic, and must be considered first in a young puppy. However, there can be other causes of a bloody stool, ones seen more in adult dogs. Following is a list of the most common ones:

Causes of Diarrhea and Their Diagnostic Tests	
Cause of Diarrhea	**Diagnostic Tests**
Viral	fever, history of exposure to other dogs, viral titers, fecal viral isolation
Bacterial	fever, bacterial cultures and sensitivity
Protozoal	lack of fever, fecal flotation test, fecal direct smear
Parasitic	fecal flotation test, fecal direct smear
Food Allergies	RAST allergy test, hypoallergenic diet trial
Dietary Indiscretion	abdominal x-rays, identification of material in feces

- Stressful situations, such as being kenneled
- Colon cancer or polyps
- Bleeding stomach ulcer with black "tarry" stools (called *melena*, which is digested blood)
- HGE (*hemorrhagic gastroenteritis*), an acute bloody diarrhea, probably due to eating inappropiate foods.
- Coprophagy (stool eating)

Constipation

Constipation is the opposite of diarrhea. In this condition, the stools become very hard and dry, and puppies can have trouble passing them. There are many causes of constipation, but they share the same mechanism. The stool material passes through the intestines and colon slower than normal, allowing more water to be absorbed from it. If the animal is dehydrated, this also contributes to the dryness of the stool. Constipation can be caused by generalized dehydration of the dog; intestinal parasites; low-fiber diet; poor-quality food; stressful situations, like being kenneled; ingesting foreign materials; anesthesia and surgery; fever; kidney disease; or diabetes.

The diagnosis of constipation is made by observing the puppy strain while defecating and producing dry, hard stools. There can even be some blood streaking of the stools from the trauma of passing them. The appropriate test must be performed to pinpoint the cause. Your veterinarian will know which test to run to rule out the different causes.

Treatment of the constipation will depend on the cause, but some basic symptomatic treatments apply in most cases. These include laxatives, such as mineral oil, to help pass the hard stool; foods higher in fiber; fiber laxatives; fluids (oral or intravenous) that correct the dehydration; and enemas or glycerine suppositories.

If the constipation becomes chronic, your veterinarian will have to check for all the previously listed causes to rule out the more serious ones. Occasional, uncomplicated constipation is nothing to worry about. We all get irregular from time to time. Watch for any other signs of digestive upsets or water changes (drinking or urinating more).

Flatulence (Excess Gas)

If your puppy passes gas once in a while, that's natural. It happens to the best of us. Frequent flatulence, however, may be a symptom of a different problem. Excess gas is often a precursor to diarrhea. Diagnosis for flatulence is very similar to that for diarrhea, and treatments for excess gas are the same as for diarrhea.

Lactose Intolerance

This is a problem people and animals share. *Lactose* is the sugar found in milk and dairy products. Some animals cannot digest it, due to a lack of the enzyme *lactase*, which breaks down the sugar into an absorbable form. The end result is stomach distress, abdominal gas and bloating, and diarrhea after eating dairy foods. This is more of a problem with people, as we tend to eat more milk products than do dogs. The simplest cure for this problem is to stop feeding your puppy dairy foods. The prognosis is *excellent* as long as you don't feed milk products.

Coprophagy (Stool Eating)

This is a problem seen in many young, small-breed dogs. Puppies under six months old often eat their own stools or those of other dogs, birds and cats. There are several theories as to why they do this. Some of the more common ones are a vitamin or mineral deficiency, starvation behavior, internal parasites and boredom. My opinion is that all are possible. Unfortunately, all vets see perfectly healthy, well-adjusted, properly fed puppies who still eat their stools. Most owners find this behavior horrifying and seek advice from their veterinarian to stop it.

It is a good idea to try to stop this bad habit because it can lead to vomiting, diarrhea and internal parasites, besides being a poor health practice. People have tried to train their dogs not to eat stool. This is very difficult, and even professional trainers become frustrated with these cases. The other measures are an attempt to make the stool very distasteful by sprinkling it with hot pepper sauce, Tabasco sauce and meat tenderizers. Increasing the fiber content of the diet also seems to help.

But don't fret too much over this problem. Most dogs outgrow this bad habit by the time they're six months old. Those who continue to do it after that age need some strong professional advice.

Anal Gland Problems

Anal glands, or sacs as they're sometimes called, are skunk-like glands all dogs have. There is one on either side of the rectum, at five and seven o'clock. The glands secrete a very smelly brown fluid that has a skunk odor every time the dog defecates. In days gone by, when dogs lived wild, these glands were scent glands. Every time the dog defecated, it excreted a small amount of this fluid, which left a lingering odor at that site. This was a means of "marking," or scenting, their territory. Our dogs still use these glands to scent their yards or sidewalks. The problem with them is they tend to get diseased, in part due to their close proximity to the rectum. Following are descriptions of the two most common disorders of the anal glands.

Anal Gland Impaction. If the secretion inside the anal glands cannot be excreted, it dries out. Instead of being a liquid, it turns into a paste or, worse, a dried-out clump that the dog can't excrete. Adding to this problem, the gland continues to secrete new liquid, resulting in a gland that is overfilled, distended, itchy and painful. What dogs do when the glands get like this is try to express them themselves, itching their rectums. Most often this behavior manifests as licking under the tail and "scooting" their bottoms on the floor. When you first observe this behavior, suspect an anal gland problem. Your veterinarian will have to express the glands manually. If the material is too hard, it may have to be softened by flushing the gland with soapy water. This breaks up the material so that it can be expressed easily. Most cooperative dogs can have this procedure done without anesthesia. Sometimes a mild sedative is needed. The prognosis is *good*, especially if you are tuned-in to the early warning signs of a problem.

Anal Gland Infection and Abscess. If a gland goes too long impacted, it becomes overdistended and damaged. It can bleed, become inflamed and get infected. The infection is common due to the close proximity to the rectum. There is a high potential for contamination. At first, the gland drips a bloody, yellow, pus discharge. The puppy usually licks at the rectal area, which is very painful. If the infection continues, the gland will *abscess* (break open to the outside) and drain the bloody

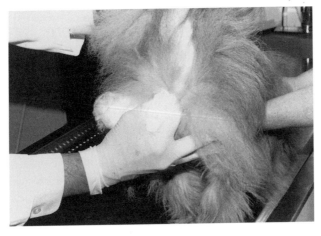

A veterinarian expresses a dog's anal glands with cotton. *Pam Koerner*

fluid described previously. After the gland abscesses, the hole left open needs to be flushed out. What I do is sedate the puppy (some need to be anesthetized), flush out the gland and the small duct (the tube that normally empties the gland), and fill it with antibiotic ointment. *It is imperative that the veterinarian flush out the gland duct also, or the gland will impact and abscess all over again.*

The puppy is then placed on oral antibiotics. Owners are asked to apply a warm compress to the area twice daily. The moist heat greatly accelerates healing. These cases generally take two to three weeks to heal fully. Unfortunately, a gland can abscess more than once. The best way to prevent anal gland abscesses is to have your veterinarian express the gland empty as soon as the dog starts showing symptoms of having rectal itching. The prognosis is *guarded* to *fair* due to the high rate of reoccurrence.

Intussusception

Intussusception is defined as the telescoping of a loop of small intestine into itself, causing an obstruction to the flow of intestinal material and fluids. Intussusception is a common sequela to ingestion of a foreign object. The object causes the intestines to contract continually in an attempt to move it through the gut. If the object doesn't move, the gut can telescope over itself, causing a worse obstruction. Affected puppies usually have bloody diarrhea, vomiting, loss of appetite and straining to defecate. Sometimes the intussusception can be felt by a rectal exam.

The difference between the treatment of an intussusception and a foreign body obstruction is that laxatives like mineral oil cannot undo the telescoped small intestine. These cases are all treated with surgery, and timing is of the essence. The loop of small intestine is manually pulled out from itself. If it has been there for more than twenty-four hours, there is a good chance that the lack of blood supply had compromised the gut, requiring its removal. This makes the surgery much more involved and makes for a *poor* prognosis.

Hormonal Disorders

Most of the hormonal problems that affect puppies were discussed in Chapter 1, since most of them are congenital defects. The diseases were juvenile diabetes mellitus, pituitary dwarfism, hypothyroidism and hypoglycemia. The one missing is *Addison's disease*, which can occur in any breed without it being inherited or congenital. Females are more prone than males.

Addison's Disease

This is a condition in which there are low levels of the body's natural cortisone. It can happen to older dogs or young puppies. Cortisone (more formally known as glucocorticoids) is secreted by the adrenal gland, which is a small gland that sits next to the kidney. Glucocorticoids are needed for maintaining the metabolism of the body's cells. Without enough, the animal will go into a state of breakdown and, ultimately, shock. Afflicted puppies are weak, have a slow heart rate and have digestive problems. They don't develop normally; they are runts and have poor coats.

Diagnosis is made by performing a basal cortisol (cortisone) level, which is a blood test. Other laboratory changes can include electrolyte imbalances, low blood sugar and anemia. The other laboratory test that can diagnose this disease is called an ACTH stimulation test, in which the patient is injected with a hormone that is supposed to stimulate cortisone production. If there are still low levels of cortisol after this, the diagnosis of Addison's disease is made.

Treatment of this disease consists of supplementing the puppy with glucocorticoids. This can be done orally or via injection. Since there are side effects to chronic glucocorticoid use, the goal is to use the lowest dose possible to manage the disease. Any breed can get Addison's disease, although some think it may be genetic in Potugese Water Dogs. The prognosis is *guarded* to *fair*.

Musculoskeletal Diseases

This section deals with the diseases and ailments that affect young, growing bones and muscles and their ligaments and tendons. It describes some of the more common traumatic injuries that can occur when a young puppy pushes its limit during play or work. We will start with injury to the muscles and end with bone trauma.

Muscle Strains, Pulls and Cramps

We have all at some point in our lives overdone an activity to the point that it caused a muscle strain or pull. Muscles are made up of many, many stringy fibers that slide over each over to form a contraction. They are highly vascular, with many arteries and veins. Nerves run through the muscles to control each and every contraction. Since each muscle fiber is a finite entity covered with a sheet of fibrous tissue, there are limits to the extent to which it can contract. When these limits are pushed or ignored, damage to the muscle fibers results. If the damage is extensive, bleeding can occur within the muscle, leading to bruising. Inflammation quickly follows the tear to the muscle fibers. Swelling and pain ensues, which can last for days to weeks.

Cramping is not as dramatic. Muscle cramps occur when there is oxygen deprivation to the muscle, or when there is a buildup of lactic acid, which is a by-product of muscle contraction. Cramps are usually temporary, lasting a minute or so. The muscle is in an involuntary contraction, which is very painful while it happens but quickly relieves itself.

Diagnosis is relatively easy in these cases. There is often a history of the puppy playing rough and suddenly coming up lame. Within the hour, there is swelling and pain of a muscle, or group of muscles. Treatment is not necessary in mild cases. In more severe ones, anti-inflammatory drugs, warm/moist compresses, and rest are needed. If a muscle is actually torn, a complete recovery can take weeks or months. The prognosis is *good*, except for very serious tears of the muscle.

Tendonitis and Tendon Strain

Tendonitis is defined as inflammation of the tendons, which are the fibrous bands that connect the muscles to bone. All muscles are connected to bones at both ends by their tendons. If enough stress is placed on the tendon, the filaments of the tendon can tear. These injuries are very common during heavy exercise or work. Any tendon is susceptible to straining. The first symptom of a strained tendon is acute pain and swelling at the site of injury. X rays will be normal since no orthopedic damage has occurred to the bone structure.

Veterinarians grade lameness in animals from 1 to 5, with 1 being barely noticeable and 5 meaning the animal won't use the leg at all. Dogs with tendonitis usually have a 1- or 2-grade lameness.

Treatment consists of applying ice packs to reduce acute swelling within the first twelve hours and using moist heat from then on. A soft padded bandage may be needed to help splint and support the damaged muscle and tendon. Resting the injury is essential for proper healing. This means staying inside, not going up or down stairs, and going outside only on a leash. Anti-inflammatory drugs like aspirin also reduce pain and swelling. The owner must abide by these rules, or the tendon will either not heal or take a very long time to heal. The prognosis is *fair* to *good* with proper rest.

Cranial Cruciate Sprain and Rupture

The cruciate ligament is the main ligament that holds the knee joint (also called a *stifle* in animals) together. The stifle is made up of three bones: the *femur* (upper leg bone), the *tibia* (the lower leg bone) and the *patella*, or knee cap. The cruciate ligament keeps the femur from sliding over the tibia bone. Large and giant breed dogs are more prone to this injury due to their size and the force they put on their joints and ligaments.

During intensive exercise or play, the dog can damage its ligament. Twisting motion is the most common way this ligament is torn. With the feet planted firmly on the ground and the upper body twisting, the cruciate ligament is at risk of injury. If the ligament is stretched or partially torn, it's called a *sprain*. There will be immediate pain in the joint. Hurt dogs do limp quite a bit, but rarely will they be "three-legged lame" (holding that hind leg up). If the dog completely ruptures the ligament, the pain will be almost unbearable and the lameness severe.

Diagnosis is made when a dog has a history of acute lameness following jumping or rough playing, or by observing a dog walk, checking for a *draw sign*, and taking an X ray. The draw sign is a technique veterinarians

Treatment Options For Cranial Cruciate Damage	
Type of Cruciate Damage	**Treatment Options**
Cruciate ligament sprain	anti-inflammatory and muscle relaxant drugs
	splints
	padded bandages
	cage rest
Complete cruciate rupture	surgery
	physical therapy and rehabilitation

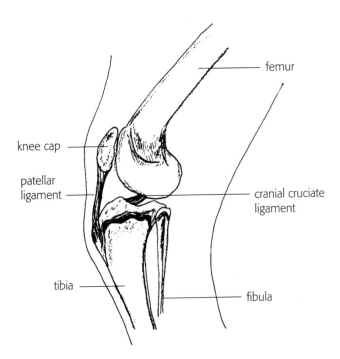

Drawing of a normal stifle (knee joint).

use to detect play or laxity in the knee joint. With the dog's knee slightly flexed, the vet tries to slide the upper femur bone over the lower tibia. If the two bones slide over one another, the draw sign is considered positive and is diagnostic for cruciate rupture. Complete ruptures of the ligament have a more dramatic draw sign. An X ray is used if a complete rupture is suspected. If the rupture is complete, the end of the torn ligament takes a small piece of bone with it. This is noticeable on the X ray and diagnostic for a complete rupture.

Treatment varies depending on whether the rupture was partial or complete. Also, different vets treat these cases differently. The above chart summarizes treatment options for both conditions.

Partial tears and ruptures generally heal without surgery. This may mean that the dog must spend weeks in a bandage or splint and have complete rest, followed by a month or two of reduced activity. The owner must abide by these rules, or the partial tear can progress to a complete rupture.

The surgery to repair a complete cruciate rupture involves reconstruction of the ligament. The joint is opened and inspected for a chipped bone fragment. If there is one, it is removed. Several different surgical techniques exist. Some surgeons utilize the patellar ligament to reconstruct the cruciate ligament. Others use man-made materials like surgical stainless-steel wire or nylon heavy-gauge suture. If done well, the surgery is an excellent way to bring the dog back to almost-100-percent recovery. The postoperative considerations are a recovery period of several weeks and a chance of arthritis developing in the knee joint months to years down the road.

Physical therapy and rehabilitation are excellent ways to get the stifle joint back into shape. Slowly building up the muscles around the joint will strengthen it. Sitting in a whirlpool, or just plain swimming, are great ways to rehabilitate a joint. The exercise is non-impact, but effective. *The key is a gradual return to function.*

The prognosis depends on the extent of the damage to the ligament. Partial ruptures, if treated correctly, carry a *fair* to *good* prognosis. Complete ruptures are more *guarded* to *fair*, even with surgery. This is due to the common occurrence of post-operative arthritis and the likelihood of concurrent cartilage damage.

Joint Swelling

Swelling of any joint can be a frustrating diagnostic challenge. What's easy to see is how painful a joint can get when it's inflamed—so painful that an animal will refuse to use the leg. Joints that are commonly afflicted are the shoulder, carpus (wrist), stifle (knee) and hock (ankle). The most common causes of joint swelling in young puppies are infectious bacterial joint disease following trauma, joint dislocation, Lyme disease (see Chapter 2), rheumatoid arthritis and systemic lupus erythematosus.

The veterinarian must figure out the cause of the swelling. Sometimes it's obvious, such as in the cases of trauma. Differentiating between infectious bacterial joint disease and Lyme disease, however, can be difficult. The autoimmune diseases (rheumatoid arthritis and lupus) are very similar and hard to tell apart. This is done with X rays and blood tests.

Once a diagnosis is made, the appropriate treatment is started immediately. Let's go through each disease and review the cause, diagnosis and treatment.

Infectious Bacterial Joint Disease

These start as trauma to the joint—for example, a bite wound. Once the joint is punctured and bacteria are introduced into the joint, an infection isn't far behind. The joint is surrounded by a capsule of tissue, appropriately called the *joint capsule*. Once the integrity of the joint capsule is broken, the bacteria have entrance into the joint fluid, where they multiply and do damage to the joint structure, cartilage and ligaments. The joint becomes swollen and painful, and there is usually a fever. The joint will not bend due to the swelling. A diagnosis is made by having the veterinarian withdraw fluid out of the joint (we call this *tapping* the joint) and culturing for bacteria. Under microscopic examination, numerous pus and blood cells appear in the joint fluid. Bacteria can also be found. Treatment consists of draining the pus and blood from the joint and administering long-term antibiotics. Anti-inflammatory drugs are given to reduce the pain and swelling. Physical therapy may be needed to restore function and flexibility to the joint. The prognosis is *guarded*, because arthritis is common after bacterial joint infections.

Joint Dislocation

If a joint dislocates, this means the bones that make up the joint go out of alignment. This usually occurs after an injury. There doesn't need to be any more external evidence: The joint becomes swollen and painful within an hour or so and does not subside with time. The dog will not place any weight on the limb, and the pain is severe enough to keep the dog from letting anyone touch the joint. Diagnosis is made by an X ray, which visualizes the dislocation. Depending on the severity of the dislocation and whether there was concurrent ligament or tendon damage, the treatment may range from a splint or cast to surgical correction. Anti-inflammatory drugs are given to reduce the pain and swelling. The prognosis is *guarded* to *poor* for ever regaining full use of the joint.

Lyme Disease

A complete description of Lyme disease is found in Chapter 2. The spirochete that causes the disease, *Borrelia burgdorferi*, invades the joints of dogs. There can be swelling and pain in the joint. There is usually a concurrent fever. The difference between this condition and the infectious bacterial joint disease is that you can rarely culture or identify the spirochete from the joint fluid. A blood test (called a *titer*) can confirm the presence of antibodies to the spirochete, which suggests a positive exposure. X rays show arthritic changes to the joint. Treatment is started as soon as Lyme disease is suspected, and involves taking antibiotics and anti-inflammatory drugs, sometimes for months.

Rheumatoid Arthritis

This is an autoimmune disease that affects all the joints of dogs (and people). For reasons unknown, the body starts an inflammation within the joint. Afflicted dogs can have fever and aches, and multiple joints can be affected. The arthritis and damage within the joint can be severe. Often, cartilage is destroyed. X rays show the damage and degenerative joint changes.

Treatment is aggressive: Anti-inflammatory drugs and cortisone are given to halt the destructive autoimmune process. Severe cases may need chemotherapy. Physical therapy, warm moist heat and walking are other treatments. These poor puppies are never normal and may be crippled by early adulthood. The prognosis is *guarded* to *poor*, even with treatment.

Systemic Lupus Erythematosus (SLE)

This disease is similar to rheumatoid arthritis in that it also is an autoimmune disease. The difference is that not only are the dog's joints affected, but so are other organ systems, like the skin and kidneys. These patients are much sicker, due to the kidney involvement. Anytime there are concurrent joint and kidney disease, SLE must be considered. Diagnosis is made by blood tests, kidney biopsy and X rays of the joints. The treatment for the arthritic portion of lupus is the same as for rheumatoid arthritis. Other measures are taken for the kidney disease as well. The prognosis is *poor*.

Fractures

A fracture is simply a broken bone. A bone can break in many different ways. Sometimes the way a bone breaks depends on the forces or strain that causes the break; sometimes it depends on where the bone breaks. The important thing to remember is that *not all breaks are the same*. Let's review the different types of fractures.

When a fracture occurs, regardless of what kind of break it is, the symptoms are pain and swelling at the site of fracture and immediate lameness, with the dog not using the leg and either letting it dangle or dragging it. There may be a crunching noise when the leg is manipulated.

Diagnosis is made by having your veterinarian palpate the leg at the site where the fracture is suspected. Ultimately, an X ray is needed to differentiate among the type of fractures. This is important, because different fractures are treated differently. Your vet will usually take two views of the leg from two different angles, to get the best picture. After reading the X rays, he or she will make recommendations as to how to treat the fracture. This may range from a padded bandage, to a cast, to surgery. Before we get into the different treatment options, let's go over some basic principles of bone healing.

In order for bones to heal, the two ends must be brought together so that they are touching each other. This is called *reduction* of the fracture. Sometimes this can be done just by manipulating the leg (called *closed* reduction). Other times it must be done surgically under anesthesia if the

Glossary of Fracture Terms

Avulsion Fracture. A fracture in which a piece of bone is pulled off where ligaments or tendons attatch.

Closed Fracture. The skin is not broken, and no bone protrudes from the limb.

Comminuted Fracture. A severe fracture that splinters and breaks into many small pieces.

Greenstick Fracture. This occurs when a young pliable bone is bowed and one side cracks, just like a twig. We see it in puppies less than six months.

Oblique Fracture. A fracture that is on a diagonal to the long bone.

Open Fracture. The fractured bone is protruding from the skin (used to be called *Compound*).

Spiral Fracture. A fracture that spirals, or curls, around the long bone.

Transverse Fracture. A fracture that is perpendicular to the long bone, all the way across.

---

muscles are contracting, to keep the two ends of the bone separated (called *open* reduction). In order to heal, the bone ends must be kept together and absolutely still. This is called *immobilization* of the fracture site. Bone ends cannot heal if there is motion. Therefore, the fracture site must be made stable by either of two means: external or internal fixation (discussed further on in this section). *External fixation* means stabilizing and immobilizing the fracture by using external means such as bandages, casts or splints. These devices keep the fracture site stable without surgery having to be performed. Padded bandages are used commonly on the lower extremities, such as the paws. Splints and casts are also used on the lower parts of the legs, either below the knee (for a hind leg) or the elbow (for a front leg). *In order for a splint or cast to work, it must immobilize the joint below and the joint above the fracture site.*

Splints and casts don't work well above the knee (for a hind leg) or elbow (for a front leg) because immobilizing the joints above the fracture is difficult. For example, let's take a fracture of the mid-humerus, or upper arm bone. When putting a splint or cast on the front arm, a veterinarian can easily include the elbow, which is the joint below the fracture line. The joint above the fracture line is the shoulder. Shoulders are almost impossible to put in a cast. This makes fractures of the humerus poor candidates for a casting or splinting. If this is done, you can expect unfavorable results.

External Fixation: Casts and Splints. These are stiff bandages that keep fractures immobile. They are best used on lower extremities of the legs. Today, most casts are either fiberglass or sectioned from prefab plastic. The advantage to fiberglass or plastic casting is that they're lightweight, waterproof and easy to apply and remove. Splints are usually made of pliable aluminum strips or rods. Casts and splints can stay on anywhere from four to twelve weeks, depending on which bone is fractured and how badly. Keeping them dry and soil-free is the hardest part. Most dogs tolerate them but may limp for a few weeks until they get used to the idea.

Internal Fixation: Hardware. When a fracture is not a good candidate for external fixation, the other alternative is internal fixation. Internal fixation is a surgical alternative. There are several different types of internal fixation. Again, the same principles apply: There has to be complete immobilization at the fracture site in order for it to heal. Examples of fractures that need internal fixation are fractures of the upper arm (humerus); fractures of the upper leg (femur); avulsion fractures; spiral fractures; fractures in dogs that can't tolerate casts; and fractures in dogs that need to recuperate quickly. The actual hardware consists of wires, screws, intramedullary pins (rods that insert down the middle of the bone shaft), bone plates, external Kirschner rods that support from the outside or a combination of these.

Internal fixation of a fracture—for example, a mid-femur transverse fracture—would involve running an intramedullary pin down the middle of the shaft in the marrow cavity. This provides side-to-side stability. One wire is placed around the shaft of the bone to add rotational stability so that, between the pin and the wire, the fracture is completely stabilized. Healing is usually swift (within eight weeks), and some of the internal hardware is left in for life.

It is beyond the scope of this book to explain all the ways fractures are repaired. Your veterinarian will have to decide which option to take for your puppy's particular fracture. In fact, some fractures don't require any fixation—internal or external. This is particularly true for fractures of the pelvis, where, depending on the location of the fracture, only cage rest is needed for a complete recovery.

Panosteitis (Growing Pains)

This is the most common non-congenital bone disorder of young dogs in the six- to eight-month age group. Dogs at high risk are the large, fast-growing breeds. The disorder happens at the age when the long bones are growing the fastest. The puppies come up lame, as there is pain associated with panosteitis. There is usually a shifting leg lameness, which means the lameness doesn't stay in the same leg but goes from leg to leg. The veterin-arian will be able to diagnose the disease by pressing on the long bones to elicit pain. Further diagnostic measures include an X ray, which shows a thickening and an inflammation of the bone. Treatment is twofold: anti-inflammatory drugs to reduce the pain, and attempts to slow down the rate of growth of the puppy. This can be accomplished by changing the diet from a puppy diet to an adult maintenance one. Also, discontinue the use of any and all vitamin and mineral supplements. Even without any treatment, the disorder resolves on its own in a couple of months as the growth rate naturally slows. The prognosis is *good*, since no permanent damage ever occurs from this condition.

Neurological Diseases

A number of congenital neurological disorders were described in Chapter 1. They included cerebellar hypoplasia, narcolepsy, vestibular disorders, GM-1 disease Wobbler's, epilepsy and laryngeal paralysis. In Chapter 2, the viral diseases canine distemper and rabies were described. These are the most common viral diseases that cause neurological symptoms in puppies. Poisonous plants and household toxins that produce neurological disease are described in Chapter 5. The diseases listed in this chapter are either traumatic or infectious in nature.

Head Trauma

Head trauma occurs most often from car accidents—for instance, a blow to the head by a tire or bumper. Dogs also experience head trauma by falling down stairs, being hit by a stick or ball (usually a baseball), running into a tree while chasing a cat, participating in dog fights and falling off ledges and hitting their heads. Regardless of the cause of the trauma, the brain responds in a similar manner: Contusion and swelling of the brain starts within minutes after severe head trauma occurs, due to an increase in pressure inside the skull. Bleeding starts next, and spaces normally filled with fluid now fill with blood, including around the brain and brain stem. Then there is edema and tissue swelling of the brain itself, and, because of all the swelling and bleeding inside the skull, the pressure gets so great that the brain actually starts to get squeezed out of the opening in the back part of the skull. This is called *herniation* of the brain, and all of it can happen without any external evidence of trauma. X rays may reveal a fractured skull, but not always.

The clinical signs of severe head trauma are unique, and you or your veterinarian would notice them shortly after the accident. Not all are seen with every case; it depends on the severity of the trauma. The more serious cases will have more of the symptoms. These are unconsciousness (being "knocked-out"), shock, rapid or slowed breathing and/or heart rate, fixed small pupils that do not react to bright light, fixed dilated pupils that do not react to bright light, flickering of the eyes in a rhythmic motion, and coma.

Treatment of head trauma depends on its severity. Mild cases may require only supportive measures for the generalized shock. These include intravenous fluids and massive doses of cortisone drugs to try to stabilize the internal bleeding. More severe cases will require releasing the pressure of the swelling and bleeding inside the skull. This is accomplished by the veterinary surgeon drilling holes at specific sites in the skull to drain the fluids. Even with this treatment, the prognosis is *poor*.

Facial Paralysis or Palsy

Facial paralysis occurs when there is trauma to the facial nerve on one side of the face. This can happen as a result of a kick or blow to the side of the head. The facial nerve is needed to keep the facial muscles toned. Without proper functioning of this nerve, the facial muscles sag and atrophy (shrink), and the eyelids droop. The lips on that side also droop. The dog presents the following facial characteristics on the side of the face with the trauma:

- A partially closed eye (which may look smaller because of the sagging eyelids)
- Excessive drooling and salivation
- Drooping eyelids and lips

Most of these traumatic facial palsy cases are temporary and resolve spontaneously. Therefore, they carry a *good* prognosis.

Spinal Cord Injuries

The spinal cord is the rope of neurologic fibers that runs from the base of the brain to the tail. It carries all the nerve impulses from the body to the

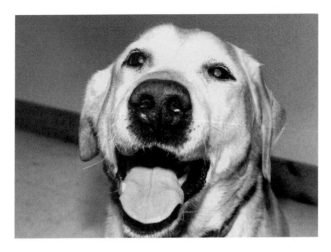

If a dog experiences trauma to the side of its face, facial paralysis may result, as seen in this dog.

brain, and vice versa. If any disruption occurs in these nerve pathways, vital information will not get through. When that happens, bodily functions stop working. This can include paralysis of a limb, the urinary bladder, the rectum and breathing.

When we talk about spinal injuries, we refer to the segment of the spinal column that is the nearest to the injury. So before you can understand spinal lesions, you must get a quick course in the spinal column. The spinal column is made up of vertebrae, which are block-like sections of bone through the center of which runs the spinal cord. The vertebrae are arranged in the following fashion:

- There are seven *cervical* (neck) vertebrae.
- There are thirteen *thoracic* (chest and ribs) vertebrae.
- There are seven *lumbar* (middle back) vertebrae.
- There are three *sacral* (lower back) vertebrae, fused into one.
- There are anywhere from one to twenty-four *coccygeal* (tail) vertebrae.

Trauma to the spinal cord can come in several different forms, as does head trauma: from being in a car accident, falling down stairs, being caught in a garage door or falling off a deck. Whether the injury is directly to the spinal cord or whether it causes the intervertebral cartilage disc's malalignment and pinches the cord, the outcome is the same. This chart offers a summary of the different types of lesions and their severity.

Varying Degrees of Spinal Cord Injuries and Their Severity		
Type of Lesion	Symptoms	Prognosis
Mild contusion and bruising	pain on movement	very good
Steady compression on cord	severe pain, can be unbearable	guarded to fair
Severed cord	loss of pain or feeling	poor

The location of the spinal lesion also helps determine the clinical symptoms. Without going into the very complex reasons why, we will give you a summary chart of what you can expect from a spinal injury based on where it is. Before we do, we need to define a few terms: *paraparesis*, a weakening of all four legs due to spinal cord contusion or compression; *paraplegia*, the complete loss of control of all four legs due to a severed spinal cord; *tetraparesis*, a weakness of the hind legs due only to spinal cord contusion or compression; and *tetraplegia*, the complete loss of control of the hind legs due only to a severed spinal cord.

When a segment of spinal cord becomes traumatized, it can behave in one of two ways. It can cause either limp paralysis or rigid stiffness of the area of the body it controlled. Whether there is paralysis or rigidity depends on which spinal fibers are disrupted. Following is a sketch of a brain, a brain stem, and the segments of a spinal cord. The abbreviations are **C** for cervical vertebrae, **T** for thoracic vertebrae, **L** for lumbar vertebrae, and **S** for sacral vertebrae. Locations are approximate.

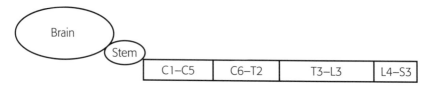

A lesion between C1 and C5 will result in all four legs being rigid, with no control.

A lesion between C6 and T2 will result in paralyzed front legs and rigid hind legs.

A lesion between T3 and L3 will result in rigid hind legs.

A lesion between L4 and S3 will result in complete paraparesis or paraplegia.

Spinal cord trauma can be diagnosed in several ways. An observant clinician will be able to examine the injured dog and localize the spinal lesion in one of the preceding situations. Many times, the exact location of the injury must be ascertained. This is especially true if surgery is the treatment of choice, in which case diagnostic X rays will need to be taken to show the vertebrae and their positions in relation to each other.

This doesn't tell you how severe the damage to the spinal cord is. To determine that, most vets take a special X ray called a *myelogram*, where a contrast dye is injected into the spinal column to outline the spinal cord on the X ray. This is a beautiful way to identify the exact spot of the spinal cord that is being pinched or impinged upon. There are a number of complications to this procedure, so discuss this option thoroughly with your vet. Other alternatives are CAT scans or MRI imaging tests. These are expensive and available only in certain locations: veterinary colleges, large referral centers and cities. Treatment of spinal cord injuries involves a few basic principles:

- Stabilization of the injured site. Great care must be taken in transporting these injured dogs.
- Reducing the swelling, inflammation and pressure on the spinal cord. This is done with anti-inflammatory drugs and surgery. If the pressure on the spinal cord is a direct result of a slipped intervertebral disc, it must be removed.
- Timing is everything. Spinal cord injuries must be treated *promptly, or irreversible cord damage will occur*. In fact, in severe cases, corrective surgery needs to be done within four to eight hours of the accident.

The prognosis varies with the type and severity of spinal cord trauma, but generally it is *poor*.

Tetanus

Tetanus is an infectious disease of the nerves and muscles of dogs (and people). The cause of this disease is a bacterium called *Clostridium tetani*. This bacterium lives in the ground and soil, especially in areas where there is manure from barnyard animals. The bacteria gain entry into tissue through deep puncture wounds. Because these bacteria cannot grow in the presence of oxygen, the wound must be deep. The bacteria inhabit tissues and secrete a neurotoxin that affects the spinal cord and brainstem. The clinical signs are complete rigidity and spasms of most of the muscles of the skeletal system. The facial and jaw muscles are usually affected first. The disease then progresses to rigidity of the leg, neck and back muscles. These poor dogs literally get as stiff as a board. They usually overreact to stimuli, such as light and noise, and symptoms can go on for weeks and months. During this time, the dog needs constant support and nursing.

These dogs should be kept quiet and in a dark room. Long-term antibiotics are given in an attempt to kill the bacteria. *Tetanus antitoxin*, an antiserum that helps bind the toxin and inactivate it, is given by injection, and tranquilizers and muscle relaxants are given to try to relieve the discomfort of the cramped muscles.

Preventing this disease means avoiding deep puncturing wounds, especially in areas with manure in the soil. If that is impossible, a vaccine of sorts is available for tetanus. It is called a *toxoid*, which means it is the attenuated tetanus toxin. Ask your veterinarian whether your puppy is at risk of contracting tetanus and whether using the toxoid is a good idea. The prognosis is *poor*.

Urogenital Diseases

Urogenital diseases are those that affect the urinary system and the genitals. This includes the kidneys and urinary bladder in both sexes, and the uterus and ovaries in females, and the testicles in the male. Chapter 1 covered some of these diseases: agenesis of the kidney, dysplasia of the kidney, ectopic ureter, hypospadias, nephropathy, patent urachus and diverticulum, polycystic kidney and urolithiasis. This section deals with the other common urogenital disorders seen in puppies under one year of age.

Renal Failure

"Renal" is another word for "kidney." If renal failure occurs suddenly, we call it acute. If the failure occurs over time, we call it *chronic*. There are several ways a young, healthy puppy's kidneys can stop working. The most common causes of kidney failure are the following: anything that reduces the blood flow to the kidneys (trauma, circulatory shock and severe blood loss), severe dehydration, anesthesia overdose, ethylene glycol (antifreeze) poisoning, ingestion of poisonous plants (such as acorns), household toxins (such as turpentine and phenol cleaners) and Lyme disease. The symptoms of acute kidney failure are varied. The majority of cases show the following symptoms: loss of appetite; vomiting and nausea; urine smell on breath; pale mucous membranes; anemia; excessive water drinking; unconsciousness; and coma.

When the veterinarian performs a blood test, the changes that are most dramatic are these:

1. The *BUN* (blood urea nitrogen) serum chemistry test is greater than 40mg/dl.

2. The *creatinine* serum chemistry test is greater than 1.5mg.

3. Urine concentration is poor, with *specific gravity* approaching that of water (less than 1.008).

4. The CBC (complete blood count) shows an anemia of a packed cell volume of less than 25 percent.

5. *Phosphorus* levels in the blood are elevated (greater than 11mg/dl).

Let's go through each of the preceding changes so that you have a better idea of what happens in kidney failure.

BUN Test. Urea nitrogen is a normal waste product of bodily function and protein metabolism. There is always a certain level of blood urea nitrogen that is considered normal; usually, it is below 40mg/dl. This number increases as the kidney function decreases, or in the presence of severe dehydration. As the urea nitrogen levels get over 60mg/dl, symptoms of kidney failure are apparent.

Creatinine. This kidney function test is considered even more accurate than the loss of BUN in diagnosing kidney failure. The reason is that this test is not generally affected by dehydration. If the results are elevated, it is quite certain that kidney failure is the cause. Anything over 1.5 is abnormal, with the more severe cases of kidney failure having numbers that range from 3.0 to 10.0.

Specific Gravity. Normally, the kidneys filter the body's blood supply, removing waste products and toxins. The kidneys also filter out water, some salts, and other bodily waste products in the urine. The urine produced should be more concentrated than water. That's what gives urine its yellow color. When the kidneys fail, they cannot concentrate the urine. The *specific gravity* is a measure of how concentrated a solution (in this case, urine) is. Normal concentrations of urine range from 1.025 to 1.040. When kidneys fail, this concentration can drop to 1.008 or less.

CBC. This stands for *complete blood count*. This blood test gives counts of the different types of blood cells. The *packed cell volume*, or *PCV*, gives a percentage of red blood cells in the blood. Normal values range from 30 to 45 percent. In cases of kidney failure, the PCV is low, usually under 30 percent. This is because the kidneys are involved in keeping a certain level of red blood cells at all times. When the kidneys fail, they aren't doing their job in stimulating red blood cell production. This accounts for the anemia seen in cases of kidney failure.

Phosphorus Levels. Phosphorus is a mineral found in many foods. Since most animals eat more phosphorus than their body needs, the remainder is excreted in the urine by the kidneys. Normal levels of phosphorus in dog blood are about 3.0 to 4.5mg/dl. If the kidneys aren't functioning properly, the levels of blood phosphorus will increase by two or three times the normal amounts. This is just another indicator of kidney failure.

Diagnosis of kidney disease is made by evaluating the preceding blood tests and other tests. Because Lyme disease is a common cause of kidney disease in young, otherwise healthy puppies, a Lyme titer may be in order. (See Chapter 2 for a complete description of Lyme disease.) X rays and ultrasounds are two other ways to evaluate kidney function. Your veterinarian will have to determine which tests are appropriate for your puppy. Unfortunately, kidney failure has very few treatment options. Dialysis machines have been experimentally used only at certain veterinary colleges. Kidney transplants are only beginning to be done at large referral practices and are very costly. Intravenous fluids can be started in an attempt to dilute the toxins that build up in the blood. Even though the fluids are not as effective as the dialysis machine, they can help reduce the BUN and creatinine levels, which makes the puppy feel better. Owners often report a temporary improvement, which means the fluid therapy may be done repeatedly.

Another form of treatment, or prevention, is to reduce the amount of protein in the puppy's diet. Protein is very stressful for kidneys to filter out of the blood. Therefore, these puppies should have a protein content in their diet under 11 percent on a dry-weight basis. Several diets on the market fit this requirement. Most causes of kidney failure in otherwise healthy puppies are reversible. Certain toxins, such as antifreeze, are not. Lyme disease can go either way. Most veterinarians who treat enough Lyme disease have lost puppies to renal complications. Your veterinarian will have to advise you on whether your puppy's case is reversible or terminal. Therefore, the prognosis is *variable*.

Cystitis

Cystitis is an inflammation of the urinary bladder caused either by an irritation (bladder stones, for example) to the bladder lining or an infection of the bladder. The former condition, bladder stones, is described in Chapter 1; this section describes infectious cystitis, meaning bladder infections caused by either bacteria or yeast.

The bacteria that often infect urinary bladders are *Escherichia coli*, *Proteus vulgaris*, *Staphylococcus aureus*, *Streptococcus*, *Klebsiella*, *Enterobacter*, and *Pseudomonas aeruginosa*. These bacteria represent some of the most common bacteria that infect animals and humans. They enter the urinary bladder via outside contamination, like sitting in feces. The bacteria make their way up the urethra and into the urinary bladder. Here are the most common reasons for infectious cystitis:

- Poor hygiene
- Urine retention (holding the urine in for too long, which is common in puppies that aren't walked frequently enough)
- Diabetes mellitus
- Urinary bladder trauma
- Bladder stones or crystals

Yeast is another organism that grows in urine. Yeast will grow anywhere there is sugar to feed on. In a normal urinary bladder, a balance exists between bacterial growth and yeast growth so that neither overpopulates nor causes disease. If the bacteria are removed, such as in a dog on long-term antibiotics for an illness, the yeast flourish in the absence of bacteria and overpopulate. An overpopulation of yeast can cause yeast cystitis. The symptoms of cystitis, regardless of whether it is bacterial or yeast, include: urinary bladder pain and cramping; burning sensation upon urination; straining to urinate, which might include crying out during urination; increased urgency or frequency of urinations; blood and pus in urine, especially in the morning; and excess protein in urine. Diagnosis of cystitis is relatively easy with three lab tests: a urinalysis test, which identifies abnormalities in the urine characteristic of cystitis; a urine culture, which identifies the bacterial or yeast organism; and a urinary bladder X ray or ultrasound, which displays the bladder stones. Ultrasound is better for this than a plain X ray, because not all bladder stones show up on a plain X ray. A special X ray called a *contrast pneumocystogram* can identify all types of bladder stones: A contrast dye is injected into the urinary bladder, followed by air, which inflates the bladder; and the contrast material highlights the inner lining of the bladder wall. A full discussion of bladder stones can be found in Chapter 1.

There are four components to treating cystitis in dogs:

1. Antibiotics to kill the bacteria.

2. Urine acidifiers to lower the pH of the urine, which inhibits bacterial and yeast growth.

3. Changing the diet to one that acidifies urine and has a low *magnesium* content.

4. Removing or dissolving any bladder stones that may be present in the urinary bladder. Large stones may need to be removed surgically; smaller stones may be dissolved by special diets. These diets are used on a short-term basis only and are available through veterinarians.

Cystitis in dogs has the potential to become a chronic disease. It tends to relapse and reoccur. There may be weeks or months between episodes. To help prevent such relapses, we make the following recommendations:

- Treat cystitis for several weeks or for a least one week after all symptoms are gone.

- Keep your puppy on low-ash and magnesium diets to prevent bladder crystals and stones.

- Encourage water-drinking, even if you have to salt the diet lightly.

- Restrict any dietary supplements that add minerals to the diet, such as bone meal, vitamins with minerals, and dark green, leafy vegetables that contain calcium and other minerals.

- Use regular urinalysis tests and/or X rays to detect early evidence of cystitis.

Female Urogenital Problems

This section outlines some of the most common female problems found in young bitches anywhere from six to twelve months of age. Each is discussed separately.

Vulvar Fold Dermatitis

The *vulva* is the opening to the vagina. Many young bitches have folds of skin on either side of the vulva due to the fact that their vulvas are small and immature. Overweight dogs have larger creases. The creases formed by these folds of skin become chafed and irritated. Add to that occasional urine scald from dribbling urine, and the skin can become almost burned. These cases are intensely itchy, so the dogs are constantly licking at themselves. If the skin is broken, a *Staphylococcus* infection is a common secondary occurrence.

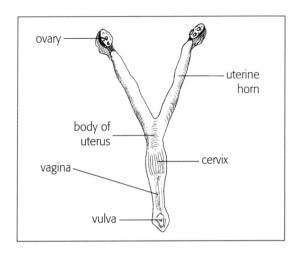

ovary

uterine
horn

body of
uterus

cervix

vagina

vulva

Drawing of the female reproductive system.

From here, the bacteria can work their way into the vagina and cause secondary vaginitis (the next disease described in this section). Classic symptoms of vulvar fold dermatitis are redness of the skin folds on either side, intense itching of the vulva, brown staining of the fur around the vulva due to excessive licking, increased urination and an infectious odor from the vulvar region.

You may notice that many of these symptoms are similar to those for vaginitis, which is described next. Diagnosis is made from external observation of the vulvar area and, perhaps, a bacterial culture to identify the causative bacteria. Treatment is similar to that for any skin infection; please refer to the part of the first section ("Skin and Coat Diseases") of this chapter entitled "Impetigo and the Staph Connection."

Puppy Vaginitis

Young bitches six to twelve months old often get inflammation and/or infection of the vagina. This is due to the fact that contamination from urine and feces is inevitable. This occurs more in sexually inactive bitches. The most common symptoms of vaginitis are redness and swelling of the vaginal mucosa (lining), a yellow pus discharge, intense itching of the vagina, excessive licking at the vulvar area, and frequent urinations and straining.

Diagnosis is made by examining the vaginal tract with a diagnostic scope. Visual inspection of the vagina will show the red, swollen lining and pus discharge. Bacterial cultures will confirm the presence of bacteria or yeast. The veterinarian may do a *vaginal smear*, which is a cotton-tipped swabbing of the vagina smeared on a microscope slide, which is then stained with a bacterial stain and examined under the microscope. The slide can show bacteria, pus cells, red blood cells and abnormal vaginal cells. All this information is valuable for the veterinarian.

The organisms grown out of a vaginal culture are frequently fecal contaminants. *Mycoplasma* is a bacterium that many breeders have been talking about recently. This organism is found deep within the vagina. To grow it out, a special culture medium is needed, so make sure your veterinarian is aware of this before sending the culture to the lab. The reason there has been much recent interest in *Mycoplasma* is because it can be a major cause of infertility later in life. A certain low level of these bacteria is considered normal, but when there is an overgrowth of them, infertility and vaginitis can result. Other bacteria that can infect the vaginal tract of young bitches are skin contaminants such as *Staphylococcus* and *Streptococcus*. Several different yeast can grow in the vaginal tract. One such yeast is *Candida*.

Chronic vaginitis (one which is present for more than a month) is a common source of infection for the urinary bladder. The bacteria can work their way up the urethra (the tube that carries the urine) and into the bladder. The preceding section on cystitis provides a complete description of the disease. Another common cause of chronic vaginitis is a congenital disorder of the ureters, which are the tubes that carry the urine from the kidney to the urinary bladder. For a complete description of this condition, see the "Ectopic Ureter" section in Chapter 1.

Treatment for vaginitis involves several measures:

1. Antibiotics for bacterial infections (topical or oral)

2. Antifungal medications for yeast infections (topical or oral)

3. Douching with antiseptic solutions

4. Topical cortisone cream to reduce itching

The prognosis is *fair* to *good* for the health of the puppy, but can be *guarded* for fertility if the vaginitis becomes chronic.

Vaginal Prolapse

This is a condition seen in young, large-breed bitches. It's observed as a red, fleshy swelling or mass protruding from the vulva that looks just like a cherry tomato. It may bleed or ooze. The mass is actually vaginal lining (mucosa) that is so swollen it has bulged out of the vagina. The cause of the vaginal tissue swelling is hormonal. When the bitch starts to go into her first heat cycle, the vaginal tissue becomes extremely swollen and may come

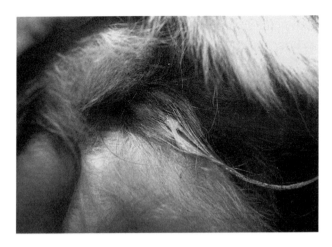

A pus discharge is a common symptom of puppy vaginitis.

out of the vagina. The bitch may have difficulty urinating around the mass of tissue.

Diagnosis is easy, as nothing else looks like a cherry tomato coming out of the vulva in a young bitch. Treatment, however, may not be so easy. If the prolapse is fresh and the tissue hasn't dried out yet, all it needs is some lubrication and it can be pushed back in. More severe cases cannot be replaced, and measures to try to reduce the swelling are needed. Ice packs can reduce the swelling, as can applying very sweet sugar solutions to the tissue, because the super-sweet sugars pull water out of tissue, shrinking it. After shrinking the tissue, the prolapse can be manually replaced with lubrication and manipulation. If the swelling is so severe that the veterinarian cannot reduce the mass, then surgery may be needed to remove it or to to suture it back in. Spaying the bitch is the best prevention if she isn't going to be used for breeding or show. Without spaying, the recurrence rate is 66 percent.

Irregular Heat Cycles

The scientific word for a heat cycle is *estrus*. This is when the bitch's ovaries start to produce the hormone *estrogen*, which is responsible for the physical changes a bitch's body goes through in preparation for breeding. The most noticeable changes are the following: the vulva swells and enlarges to accept a male; the uterus engorges, preparing for a possible pregnancy; there is a bloody vaginal discharge that attracts the male; the vaginal lining becomes swollen in preparation for breeding; and behavioral changes occur that promote breeding.

The normal bitch cycles about every six or seven months. Each heat cycle may last from one to three weeks. During that time, she will accept a male, and she will *ovulate*, meaning eggs will be released for fertilization. This is an oversimplification, because heat cycles involve a complex series of changing hormones and bodily processes that allow for breeding and pregnancy. Breeders must familiarize themselves with these so that they can help time a bitch for breeding and increase the chances of conception.

Some bitches do not have normal heat cycles. If the interval between heat cycles (called the *interestrous period*) is shorter or longer than six to seven months, we consider that abnormal. Here are descriptions of the most common abnormal heat situations:

Ovarian Cysts

If a bitch cycles more than every six months, she may have ovarian cysts. These are cysts of the ovarian tissue that produce the estrogen hormone, keeping a high level of hormone present most of the time. Diagnosis is made by running blood estrogen levels and visualizing the cysts on an ultrasound scan. The easiest way to correct this problem is to spay the bitch.

Silent Heats

If a young bitch is a year old and hasn't appeared to have her first heat cycle yet, there is a good chance you missed a very light cycle. Such cycles are shorter than normal, and there is little in the way of external evidence. The vulva may not swell, and little bleeding may occur. The whole heat may be over in a few days. Most of the bitches that have silent heats don't ovulate, so the chances that they could have bred or been impregnated are quite slim. Usually their next heat is normal.

Split Heats

These are common in small-breed bitches. In these cases, the bitch starts coming into heat, stops, and then starts up again several weeks later. The problem with this condition is that it is very difficult to time breeding, since ovulation may occur during either part, or not at all. These bitches should be spayed, as they make poor breeders. Split heats often mean that some other problem is going on.

Hypothyroidism

Hypothyroidism is a condition in which the thyroid gland produces too little thyroid hormone. (A complete description is given in Chapter 1 under "Hormonal Defects.") A low thyroid hormone level can cause irregular heat cycles and infertility in the bitch. Diagnosis is made by a thyroid hormone blood level test. Treatment is relatively easy: thyroid supplements in tablet form.

Imperforate Hymen

The *hymen* is a thin veil of tissue that blocks off the entrance to the vaginal canal in a young developing puppy. This tissue is stretched and easily broken down, such as during the first mating of a virgin bitch. It may also break down during the first heat cycle. If it doesn't, it is an impediment to natural breeding. The veterinarian may be able to break the thin diaphragm of tissue manually with an internal vaginal exam. If not, surgery may be required to remove the excess tissue.

Brucellosis

This is a contagious venereal disease of breeding dogs and bitches. It is described under "Male Urogenital Problems," as males are more prone to the disease.

Male Urogenital Problems

The male genitalia are prone to certain problems that involve either the testicles or the penis and its sheath (called the *prepuce*). The prostate is the other male urogenital organ that has frequent trouble, but we see more of that in older dogs. Each condition is described separately in this section. More of these problems occur in sexually active dogs, although any dog can get most of these conditions.

Orchitis

Orchitis means inflammation of the *testicle*, the male gonad that manufactures sperm. Normally, two testicles are suspended in the sac of skin called the *scrotum*. If there is only one, the condition is called *cryptorchidism*, a description of which is found in Chapter 1. There are three common causes of a swollen testicle in the young dog:

1. *Trauma.* Any kind of blunt trauma to the testicle will result in inflammation, pain and swelling. If the trauma is severe enough, bruising and bleeding can occur within the testicle, called a *testicular hematoma*. The swelling is transient. Ice packs and anti-inflammatory drugs can help reduce the swelling and pain. Buffered aspirin is a good all-purpose anti-inflammatory for such cases. If the testicle is damaged beyond healing, neutering is the best alternate treatment.

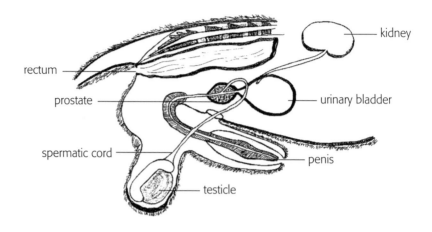

Drawing of the male reproductive system.

2. **Testicular Torsion.** As the name implies, this is when a testicle twists on itself, rotating ninety to 180 degrees inside the scrotum and shutting off the blood supply to the testicle, which causes acute swelling and intense pain in the testicle. The large and giant breed dogs are more prone to this condition. The treatment of choice is emergency neutering. If the dog is a valuable breeding stud, the veterinarian may attempt to save the testicle with emergency surgery to untwist the testicle. If it was twisted for too long (several hours), irreparable damage from lack of blood flow will occur. The veterinarian will be able to determine by looking at the testicle during surgery whether it is salvageable. If not, the other testicle may be spared.

3. **Infectious Orchitis.** Dogs can get an infection of the testicle and its associated structures (such as the epididymis) and tubes. There are two common ways a testicle can become infected: either from contamination from bacteria (fecal and skin) or from venereal diseases. Fecal bacteria can easily make their way into the testicle via the vast array of tubing that connects the penis with the testicles. The bacteria that are often cultured from semen samples of dogs with orchitis are *Escherichia coli*, *Proteus vulgaris*, *Streptococcus*, *Brucella canis*, *Staphylococcus* and *Mycoplasma*.

Brucellosis

Brucellosis is the most common sexually transmitted venereal disease. The bacterium that causes this disease is *Brucella canis*. This bacterium can cause an infection of the genitals of both males and females. The bacteria are passed from dog to bitch, or vice versa, during breeding. It infects both the male and female genital tracts, causing disease and infertility. Females don't conceive, and males have affected sperm quality. This bacterium is highly contagious in vaginal secretions, sperm and urine of infected dogs. It is also a human health hazard, as people can become infected with the bacteria, causing a serious illness.

The diagnosis is made with a blood brucella titer test, which identifies the carriers and infected individuals. Infection is treated with high doses of long-term antibiotics. In some cases, the dog is euthanized because of the possibility of human exposure.

Scrotal Dermatitis

As the name implies, this is a dermatitis of the skin of the scrotum. These are very common in young males, which are prone to licking themselves. Most often, the dermatitis starts as an insect bite or a scrape. Once the sensitive skin of the scrotum is irritated, it becomes itchy, at which point the dog licks incessantly at it, causing a worse irritation, or lick sore. The top layers of skin are licked away, exposing the dermis of the skin underneath. These may bleed, and they usually become infected with *Staphylococcus* bacteria. A local hive or welt develops, and the dog itches and scratches even more.

Treatment usually includes antibiotics and/or topical anti-inflammatory drugs. It's important to keep the dog from scratching or licking at the wound, or it won't heal. In severe cases, injections of cortisone will temporarily relieve the itch. Since bandaging a scrotum is impossible, an Elizabethan collar will keep the dog from getting to it. The essentials to treating a scrotal dermatitis are antibiotics for the infection, anti-inflammatory drugs and anti-itch (such as cortisone) to calm the itch and reduce the pain and swelling, and an Elizabethan collar to keep to puppy from making it worse. A severe case may take a few weeks to heal. With proper care, however, these conditions generally heal, carrying a *good* prognosis.

Paraphimosis

Paraphimosis is a condition in which the opening of the penis sheath is too small, making it difficult for an erect penis to retract back inside because the small sheath size causes it to roll in while the penis retracts. In most cases, the penis cannot retract fully, a condition that can be very uncomfortable for the dog. In the mild cases, a light lubricant such as petroleum jelly or mineral oil is enough to get the penis to retract. In severe cases, surgery must be performed to enlarge the prepuce opening. This is most important in breeding dogs.

Prostatitis

Prostatitis is the inflammation of the *prostate gland*. The prostate is a walnut-shaped, spongy gland needed for producing fluid for the semen. As dogs become middle-aged, there is the chance that the prostate gland will become enlarged. Since this is primarily a puppy book, we will discuss the infection of the prostate gland in young dogs only, called *prostatitis*. The same bacteria that can cause orchitis or cystitis, as described previously, can infect the prostate gland because the urinary bladder, testes and prostate gland are all connected. Symptoms of dogs with prostatitis are similar to those for cystitis. Careful diagnostic work is needed to differentiate between the two. The major difference is that the prostate gland feels enlarged on a rectal exam. The most common symptoms of prostatitis are blood in the urine, straining to urinate, pus in the urine, lower abdominal pain and a grossly enlarged prostate gland on rectal exam.

Diagnosis is made by performing the same sort of tests done to diagnose cystitis (see that section).

If the dog is a valuable breeding stud, prostatitis can be treated using long-term antibiotics. Many veterinarians choose a sulfur-type antibiotic because it gets into the urogenital tract in high concentrations. The dog is not allowed to breed for several months following prostatitis due to the accompanying poor semen quality.

If the dog is not a breeding animal, then the best cure for any prostatic disease is neutering. Once the dog is castrated, the prostate gland shrinks down to a nubbin and the infection clears up, never to return again. This is because the prostate needs the hormone testosterone to maintain its size and function, which the testes produce. Once the testes are removed, testosterone levels drop to zero, and the prostate gland can no longer maintain its function. A nonexistent gland cannot become infected.

Signs and Symptoms by Disease

Addison's Disease

Diarrhea

Exercise Intolerance

Heart Rate Decrease

Inappetence

Shock

Weakness

Allergic Dermatitis (Atopy)

Excess Tearing

Hair Loss

Hives

Inflammation

Itching

Pyoderma

Rash

Swelling

Wheal

Anal Gland Problems

Bloody Discharge

Fever

Licking at Rectum

Painful Swelling

Pus Discharge

Rectal Itching

Scooting

Anaphylaxis

Blood Pressure
  Decrease

Circulatory Shock

Death, Sudden

Lung Fluid

Aural Hematoma

Blood Clot

Egg-sized Swelling

Head Shaking

Itching

Painful Ear

Red Ear

Bacterial Otitis Externa

Crusting in Ear

Head Shaking

Infectious Odor

Inflamed Ear

Itching

Painful Ear

Pus Discharge

Red Ear

Scratching at Ear

Bee Stings and Bug Bites

Death, Sudden

Pain at Bite

Redness at Bite

Swelling at Bite

Bleeding

Arterial Bleeding

Blood Ooze

Blood Spurts

Capillary Bleeding

Hemorrhage

Venous Bleeding

Bloat and Dilatation-Volvulus

Abdominal Bloating

Diarrhea

Distended Abdomen

Doubled-over

Dry Heaving

Heart Arrhythmia

Heart Rate Increase

Hunched-over

Inflated Abdomen

Painful Abdomen

Pale Mucous
  Membranes

Rapid Breathing

Salivation

Sudden Death

Vomiting

Weak Pulse

Weakness

Bordetella bronchiseptica

Dry Hacking Cough

Fever

Goose-Honking

**Borreliosis
(Lyme Disease)**

Arthritis
Body Aching
Bull's-eye Rash
Fever
Inappetence
Kidney Failure
Lameness
Lump
Myocarditis
Paralysis
Seizures
Swollen Joints

Broken Nails

Bleeding
Painful Toe
Quick Exposed
Swelling of Toe

Bronchitis/Pneumonia

Coughing
Exercise Intolerance
Fever
Gagging
Inappetence
Labored Breathing
Laryngitis
Wheezing

Burns

Blackened Skin
Blistering
Inflamed Skin
Melted Skin
Red Skin

Calcium Deficiency

Bone Deformity
Skeletal Deformity

Callus

Dry Skin
Flaky Skin
Hair Loss
Raised Thickened
  Skin

**Canine Adenovirus
Type-1 (Infectious
Hepatitis)**

Abdominal Pain
Corneal Edema
  (Blue Eye)
Fever
Inappetence
Jaundice
Liver Swelling
Vomiting

**Canine Adenovirus
Type-2**

Coughing
Eye Discharge
Labored Breathing
Nasal Discharge
Sneezing
Wheezing

Canine Babesiosis

Anemia
Enlarged Spleen
Fever
Jaundice
Pale Mucous
  Membranes

Canine Coronavirus

Bloody Stool
Diarrhea
Fetid Diarrhea
Fever
Vomiting

Canine Distemper

Blindness
Circling
Conjunctivitis
Coughing
Dehydration
Diarrhea
Falling Over
Fever
Labored Breathing
Pneumonia
Pus Discharge
Seizures
Sneezing
Tremors
Vomiting
Weight Loss

Canine Ehrlichiosis

Anemia
Bleeding
Edema of Legs
Fever
Thrombocyte
  Deficiency

Canine Parainfluenza

Coughing
Fever
Nasal Discharge
Sneezing

Canine Parvovirus

Abdominal Pain
Bloody Stool
Explosive Diarrhea
Fetid Diarrhea
Fever

Carbohydrate Deficiency

Constipation
Hypoglycemia
Low Energy
Poor Digestion

Chalazion

Eyelid Irritation
Itching
Meibomian Gland
  Swelling
Painful Swelling
Redness of Eyelid

Choking

Coughing
Cyanosis
Death, Sudden
Fainting
Gasping
Heaving

Coccidia

Abdominal Bloating
Bloody Stools
Colitis
Diarrhea
Malnutrition
Vomiting
Weight Loss

Constipation

Blood in Stool
Dehydration
Hard Stool
Straining to Defecate

Copper Deficiency

Anemia
Coat Color Change

Corneal Ulcer

Blindness
Corneal Cloudiness
Corneal Erosion
Excess Tearing
Itching
Painful Eye
Red Eye
Squinting

Cracked Nails

Bleeding
Brittle Nails
Nail Peeling
Painful Toe

Cranial Cruciate Sprain or Rupture

Click in Knee
Pain of Knee
Swelling of Knee
Three-Legged Lame

Cropped Ears

Blood Oozing at
  Skin Margin
Itching
Scabbing

Cuts, Scrapes and Excoriations

Hair Loss
Oozing
Redness and
  Swelling

Cystitis

Bloody Urine
Burning Sensation
  on Urination
Crystals in Urine
Increased Frequency
  of Urination
Increased Thirst
Painful Urinary
  Bladder
Painful Urination
Protein in Urine
Pus in Urine
Straining to Urinate

Diarrhea and Colitis

Abdominal Pain
Bloody Stool
Dark Stool
Fever
Flatulence
Greasy Stool
Loose Stool
Melena
Mucous in Stool
Smelly Diarrhea
Straining to Defecate
Vomiting
Watery Stool
Weight Loss

Dry Eye

Brown Coating to
Eye
Corneal Ulceration
Itching
Painful Eye
Pus Discharge
Red Eye
Squinting

Ear Mites

Brown Waxy Ear
Discharge
Coffee Ground
Discharge
Crusting and Flaking
Itching
Scratching Ears
Shaking Head

Electrocution

Blackened Mouth
Circulatory Collapse
Death, Sudden
Salivation
Unconsciousness

Eyelid Infection

Closed Eye
Excess Tearing
Eyelid Irritation
Pus Discharge
Redness of Eyelid
Swelling of Eyelid
Whiteheads

Facial Paralysis

Drooped Eyelids
Drooped Lips

Facial Palsy
Partially Closed Eye
Salivation

Fat Deficiency

Dermatitis
Dull Brittle Coat
Flaky Skin
Pansteatitis

Fleas

Crusting
Flea Bite Dermatitis
Hair Loss
Itching
Red Skin
Scratching
Wheal

Fly Bites

Bleeding at Bite
Itching at Bite
Red and Painful at
Bite
Swelling at Bite
Wheal and Hive at
Bite

Foreign Object Gastroenteritis

Abdominal Pain
Coughing
Dry Heaving
Gagging
Hunched Over
Pale Mucous
Membranes
Salivation
Vomiting

Fractures

Bone Protrusion
Crunching Noise
Dangling Limb
Deviation of Limb
Lameness
Pain
Swelling

Frostbite

Line of Demarcation
Loss of Feeling
Red and Painful
Swelling

Giardia

Abdominal Bloating
Diarrhea
Mucous in Stools
Poor-Doer
Weight Loss

Head Trauma

Coma
Dilated Fixed Pupils
Flickering Eye
Movements
Heart Rate Increase
Knocked-out
Rapid Breathing
Shock
Sudden Death
Unconsciousness

Heartworm Disease

Abdominal Fluid
Cough
Dilated Pulmonary
Blood Vessels

Exercise Intolerance
Kidney Failure
Weakness
Weight Loss

Heat Stroke

Coma
Death, Sudden
Fainting
Heart Rate Increase
Panting
Ruddy Mucous
  Membranes
Salivation
Weakness

Histiocytoma

Dime-Sized Swelling
Hair Loss
Itching
Round Swelling

Hookworms

Abdominal Bloating
Anemia
Cough
Diarrhea
Dry and Brittle Coat
Emaciation
Excess Gas
Increased Appetite
Poor-Doer

Horner's Syndrome

Facial Palsy
Protruded Nictitans
  Eyelid
Smaller Pupil
Sunken Eyeball

Hot Spots and Pyoderma

Bleeding
Bull's-eye
Hives
Itching
Ulcerated Skin
Wheal

Household Substance Poisoning

Abdominal Pain
Acidic Breath
Anemia
Bleeding
Blindness
Bloody Urine
Burns
Coma
Cyanosis
Incoordination
Death, Sudden
Depression
Dilated Pupils
Disorientation
Dullness
Heart Arrhythmia
Kidney Failure
Labored Breathing
Muscle Twitching
Nausea
Rigid Muscles
Salivation
Seizures
Shock
Skin Blisters
Skin Irritation
Spasms
Urine Discoloration

Weak Pulse
Weakness

Impetigo

Itching
Open Sores
Pimples
Pyoderma
Rash
Red Skin
Scratching
Whiteheads

Ingrown Nails

Bloody Discharge
Infectious Odor
Painful Toe
Pus Discharge
Swelling of Toe

Intussusception

Abdominal Pain
Bloody Stool
Fever
Straining to Defecate
Vomiting
Weight Loss

Iodine Deficiency

Goiter
Hypothyroidism

Iron Deficiency

Anemia

Irregular Heat Cycles

Behavioral Changes
Bloody Vaginal
  Discharge

Cycle Interval
  Longer Than
  Six Months
Cycle Interval
  Shorter Than
  Six Months
Cycle Longer Than
  Two Weeks
Cycle Shorter Than
  Two Weeks
Infertility
Two Cycles Back to
  Back
Uterus Engorgement
Vulva Swelling

Joint Swelling

Aching
Arthritis
Fever
Painful Joint
Pitting Edema
Red Joint
Swollen Joint

Kidney Failure

Anemia
Coma
Excessive Water
  Intake
Inappetence
Increased Urination
Nausea
Pale Mucous
  Membranes
Sudden Death
Unconsciousness
Urine Odor of
  Breath
Vomiting

Lactose Intolerance

Abdominal Bloating
Abdominal Pain
Diarrhea
Flatulence
Stomach Distress

Laryngitis

Absence of Bark
Change in Bark
Coughing
Gagging
Stridor
Wheezing

Leptospirosis

Abdominal Pain
Bloody Stool
Body Aches
Inappetence
Jaundice
Liver Swelling
Nosebleeds
Uveitis
Vomiting

Lice

Anemia
Hair Loss
Itching
Scratching

Lick Granuloma

Hair Loss
Itching
Painful
Quarter-sized
  Swelling
Raised Thickened
  Skin

Ulcerated

**Lysosomal Storage
Disease**

Weakness
Tremors
Paralysis
Seizures

Magnesium Deficiency

Bone Deformity
Joint Deformity
Neurological
  Changes

Manganese Deficiency

Joint Deformity
Tendon Deformity

Mange

Baldness
Dandruff
Fever
Furunculosis
Hair Loss
Intense Itch
Intense Scratching
Itching
Peripheral Lympha-
  denopathy
Pyoderma
Red Patches
Scaling
Seborrhea

Motion Sickness

Drooling
Nausea
Vomiting

Muscle Sprains, Pulls and Cramps

Bruising
Inflammation
Lameness
Muscle Cramping
Pain
Swelling

Orchitis

Decreased Sperm
  Count
Fever
Infertility
Testicular Hematoma
Testicular
  Inflammation
Testicular Pain
Testicular Swelling
Testicular Torsion

Panosteitis

Growing Pains
Inflammation of
  Bone
Lameness
Long Bone Pain
Thickening of Bone

Papillomatosis

Cauliflower Growth
Clusters of Growths
Gray-colored Skin
Warts

Paraphimosis

Bleeding
Excessive Licking
Lameness

Painful Penis
Swollen Prepuce

Paronychia

Crusting
Itching
Loose Nail
Pus Discharge
Red and Painful Toe
Swelling

Pemphigus

Bleeding
Crusting
Hair Loss
Inflammation
Itching
Red Skin
Skin Blisters
Skin Exfoliation
Ulceration

Phosphorus Deficiency

Bone Deformity
Increased Appetite
Skeletal Deformity

Poisonous Plants

Abdominal Cramps
Abdominal Pain
Blood Pressure Drop
Coma
Death, Sudden
Depression
Diarrhea
Dilated Pupils
Dry Mouth
Hallucinations
Heart Arrhythmia

Increased Heart Rate
Kidney Failure
Labored Breathing
Mouth Blisters
Nausea
Numbing of Mouth
Pharyngitis
Salivation
Shock
Swallowing
Swollen Tongue
Vomiting

Potassium Deficiency

Heart Arrhythmia
Neurological
  Changes
Weakness

Proptosis

Blindness
Eye out of Socket
Painful Eye
Red Eye

Prostatitis

Abdominal Pain
Bloody Urine
Dribbling Urine
Enlarged Prostate
Fever
Frequent Urinations
Poor Urine Stream
Pus in Urine
Straining to Urinate

Protein Deficiency

Dull Brittle Coat
Leg Swelling
  (Edema)

Low Energy
Muscle Atrophy

Puppy Strangles

Bleeding
Facial Swelling
Itching
Peripheral Lympha-
  denopathy
Pus Discharge
Swollen Eyes

Puppy Vaginitis

Blood in Urine
Burning Sensation
  on Urination
Frequent Urination
Itching
Licking at Vagina
Redness of Vagina
Yellow Pus Discharge

Rabies

Aggression
Behavioral Changes
Blindness
Circling
Death, Sudden
Fever
Foaming at Mouth
Incoordination
Jaw Paralysis
Seizures
Voice Change

Retinal Detachment

Blindness
Blood in Eye
Detached Retina

Rhinitis

Fever
Itchy Nose
Photophobia
Red Eyes
Runny Eyes
Runny Nose
Sneezing
Yellow Pus Nasal
  Discharge

Ringworm

Circular Lesion
Crusting
Hair Loss
Itching
Red Skin

**Rocky Mountain
Spotted Fever**

Bloody Stool
Bloody Urine
Bruising
Diarrhea
Fever
Labored Breathing
Nose Bleeds
Rash
Vomiting

Roundworms

Abdominal Bloating
Bloody Stools
Cough
Diarrhea
Dry and Brittle Coat
Emaciation
Excess Gas
Increased Appetite

Uveitis
Vomiting
Worms in Stool

Scrotal Dermatitis

Bleeding
Excessive Licking
Irritated Scrotum
Itching
Lick Sore
Painful Scrotum
Redness

Selenium Deficiency

Muscle Atrophy
Muscle Degeneration

Shock

Blood Pressure
  Decrease
Collapse
Coma
Death, Sudden
Dilated Pupils
Disorientation
Fainting
Fixed Pupils
Heart Rate Increase
Rapid Breathing
Unconsciousness

Sinusitis

Choking
Congested Nose
Coughing
Fever
Gagging
Headache
Post-nasal Drip

Sneezing

Squinting

Yellow Pus Nasal
  Discharge

Snake Bite

Bruising

Coma

Death, Sudden

Disfigurement at Bite

Fang Holes

Neurological
  Changes

Seizures

Swelling at Bite

Spinal Cord Injury

Limp Legs

Paralysis of Legs

Stiffness in Front
  Legs

Weakness in Four
  Legs

Weakness in Front
  Legs

Weakness in Hind
  Legs

Stye

Eyelid Irritation

Itching

Painful Swelling

Redness of Eyelid

Zeis Gland Swelling

Tapeworms

Digestive Upsets

Increased Appetite

Rectal Itching

Segments in Stool

Weight Loss

Tendonitis

Inflammation

Lameness

Pain

Swelling

Tetanus

Complete Rigidity of
  Limbs

Involuntary Muscle
  Contractions

Lockjaw

Spasms

Tonsillitis

"Strep" Throat

Coughing

Enlarged Cervical
  Lymph Nodes

Enlarged Tonsils

Gagging

Infectious Odor from
  Throat

Painful Tonsils

Red Tonsils

Sore Throat

Uveitis

Blindness

Blood in Eye

Cloudy Eye

Excess Tearing

Increased Eye
  Pressure

Painful Eye

Red Eye

Squinting

Vaginal Prolapse

Bleeding

"Cherry Tomato"

Excessive Licking at
  Vulva

Increased Frequency
  of Urinations

Itching

Painful Urination

Protruding Mass
  from Vulva

Pus Discharge

Red Fleshy Swelling

Vitamin A Deficiency

Blindness

Dull and Brittle Coat

Poor Skin

Retinal
  Degeneration

Vitamin B Deficiency

Anemia

Convulsions

Inappetence

Neck Contortion

Poor Digestion

Weakness

Weight Loss

Vitamin C Deficiency

Immunosuppression

Scurvy

Vitamin D Deficiency

Bone Deformity

Rickets

Teeth Defects

Vitamin E Deficiency

Muscle Atrophy
Muscle Weakness
Pansteatitis

Vitamin K Deficiency

Bleeding
Hemophilia
Nosebleeds
Prolonged Clotting
Times

Vulvar Fold Dermatitis

Brown Staining of
Fur Around Vulva
Increased Urinations
Infectious Odor
Itching

Licking at Vulva
Redness of Vulva

Water Deficiency

Dehydration
Dry Mouth and
Gums
Weight Loss

Whipworms

Abdominal Bloating
Abdominal Cramps
Bloody Stools
Diarrhea
Dry and Brittle Coat
Excess Gas
Increased Appetite
Mucous in Stools
Poor-Doer

Yeast Otitis Externa

Brown Wax
Discharge
Crusting in Ear
Head Shaking
Inflamed Ear
Itching
Painful Ear
Red Ear
Scratching at Ear
Sour Odor

Zinc Deficiency

Baldness
Flaky Dry Coat
Seborrhea

General Index

Heartworm Disease
106–113
Heartworm Prevention
108–111
daily (diethylcarba-
mazine)
monthly (ivermectin,
milbemycin oxime)
Heartworm Treatment
110
dithiazanine iodide
thiacetarsamide
Heartworm Test 110
direct blood smear
micropore filter
modified Knott's
occult antigen
Heat Cycle, see *Estrus*
Heat Stroke 178
Heimlich Maneuver 180
Hematoma 212
Hemophilia 33
Hemorrhage, see *Bleeding*
Hemorrhagic Gastroenter-
itis (HGE) 228
Hepatic Encephalopathy
25
Hepatitis 24
Herbal Insect Repellents
87
brewer's yeast
citronella
eucalyptus
garlic cloves
menthol
Hermaphrodite 3
Herniorrhaphy 28
Hip Dysplasia 44
Histamine 184
Histamine Shock 184
Histiocytoma 199
Hive 192
Holistic Medicine 161
Homeopathy 161
Hookworm 99–102
Hormones 232
Horner's Syndrome 205
Hot Spot 192
Household Toxins
172–175

acetone
ammonia
antifreeze
aspirin
bleach
carbon monoxide
charcoal lighter
chocolate
deodorant
detergent
furniture polish
gasoline
kerosene
lead
lime
lye
organophosphate
insecticide
paint thinner
phenol cleaner
rat poison
rubbing alcohol
soap
strychnine
turpentine
Tylenol
Human Chorionic
Gonadotropin (HCG)
30
Hydatid Cyst 106
Hydrocephalus 4
Hydrogen Peroxide 171
Hydroxyurea 32
Hymen, see *Imperforate Hymen*
Hyperthermia, see *Heat Stroke*
Hypoallergenic diets 196
Hypoglycemia 21
Hypospadias 53
Hypothermia 178
Hypothyroidism 36, 254
Hypotrichosis 6

I

Idiopathic Epilepsy, see
Epilepsy
Imperforate anus 3
Imperforate hymen 255

Inappetence 218
Infertility 157
Ingredients 143
Ingrown nails 132
Inguinal hernia 7
Inguinal ring 159
Injection Techniques 61
intramuscular
intranasal
subcutaneous
Inner Ear 13
Insect Growth Regulators
85
fenoxycarb
methoprene
Insecticides 80–90
Insulin 23
Insulin Dependent 23
Insulin Non-dependent
23
Insulin Shock 23
Interestrous Period 254
Intersex, see *Hermaphrodite*
Intestinal Obstruction
231
Intestine 231
Intussusception 231
Ipecac Syrup viii
Iris 208
Iris Cyst 16
Irregular Heat Cycle 253
Isospora, see *Coccidia*
Ivermectin 108

J

Jaundice 24
Joint Capsule 236
Joint Swelling 236
bee sting
dislocation
Joint Tapping 237
Juvenile Cataract 16
Juvenile Diabetes mellitus
22

K

Kennel Cough, see
Bordetella bronchiseptica